Physical Therapy and Massage for the Dog

Julia Robertson and Andy Mead

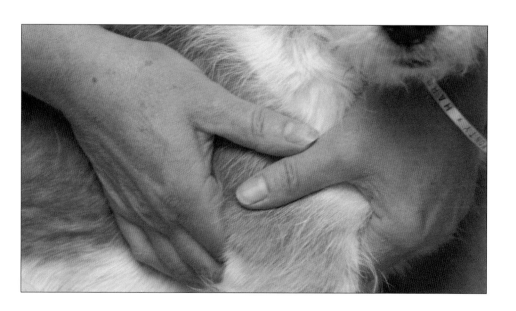

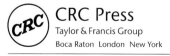 CRC Press
Taylor & Francis Group
Boca Raton London New York

CRC Press is an imprint of the
Taylor & Francis Group, an **informa** business

CRC Press
Taylor & Francis Group
6000 Broken Sound Parkway NW, Suite 300
Boca Raton, FL 33487-2742

© 2013 by Taylor & Francis Group, LLC
CRC Press is an imprint of Taylor & Francis Group, an Informa business

No claim to original U.S. Government works

Printed on acid-free paper
Version Date: 20161018

International Standard Book Number-13: 978-1-84076-144-3 (Hardback)

Visit the Taylor & Francis Web site at
http://www.taylorandfrancis.com

and the CRC Press Web site at
http://www.crcpress.com

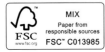

Printed in the United Kingdom
by Henry Ling Limited

Contents

Preface

This book is intended for canine physical and massage therapists, veterinary nurses, trainers, hydrotherapists, and other professionals connected with veterinary referral. The level and content could also be appropriate for informed dog owners who are keen to learn more about what is under their dog's skin.

Currently, canine massage and physical therapy are growing markets within the UK, with agility being one of the fastest growing sports. The demand is great for resource material to cover this subject, especially one from both a veterinary and specialist canine sports physical therapist perspective. The book includes case studies, sequential photographs depicting movement, detailed diagrams to demonstrate the topic, and clear methods of depicting and describing muscle position and actions.

Acknowledgements

Sincere thanks to the dogs and their owners who kindly agreed to their inclusion in this book: Copper, Dexter, Digby, George, Jess, Monty, Tally, Tia, Tiggi, Lisa Bishop, Jasper Bolton, Archie Govier, C. Kisko, Oscar Norgate, Lezleigh Packer, Archie, Alfie, Lexy, and Liz Pope, Yogi Tucker; thanks also to Henry Robertson for additional photographs.

Abbreviations

ACh acetyl choline
ADP adenosine diphosphate
ANS autonomic nervous system
ATP adenosine triphosphate
CDRM chronic degenerative
radiculo-myelopathy
CNS central nervous system
CT computed tomography
DJD degenerative joint disease
GSD German Shepherd dog
GTO Golgi tendon organ
HD hip dysplasia
LCPD Legg–Calvé–Perthes disease
LMN lower motor neuron
MRI magnetic resonance imaging

NMJ neuromuscular junction
NSAID nonsteroidal anti-inflammatory
drug
OA osteoarthritis
OCD osteochondritis dissecans
OTC over-the-counter (medication)
PNS peripheral nervous system
POM prescription-only medication
PPS pentosan polysulphate
TCM traditional Chinese medicine
TFL tensor fascia lata
TPLO tibial plateau levelling
osteotomy
UMN upper motor neuron

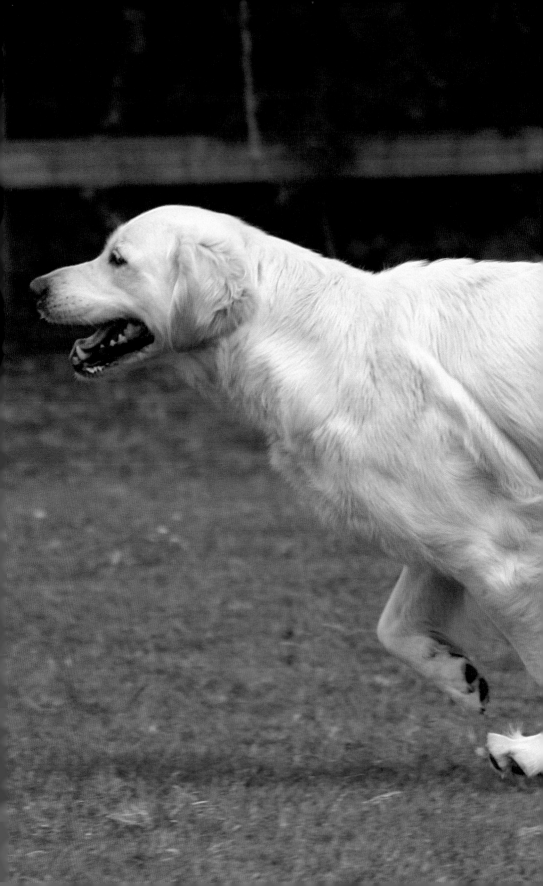

1

Introduction to Physical Therapy and Massage

Julia Robertson and Andy Mead

- Introduction
- A brief history of massage
- Current practice

Introduction

Physical therapy is concerned with the prevention, management, and treatment of movement and allied disorders. It encompasses detailed assessments and treatment programmes that involve hands-on therapy, along with dynamic remedial and strengthening techniques using exercise plans. As far as dogs are concerned, this is an evolving therapy (1), but one that has been used for centuries. It was expounded by a famous Greek practitioner, Arrian, who wrote about how massage would help horses and dogs, asserting that it would 'strengthen the limbs, render the hair soft and glossy, and cleanse the skin'.

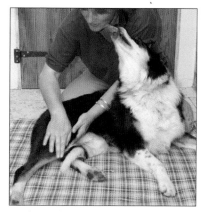

1 Physical therapy in the dog. (Courtesy of Henry Robertson.)

Medical breakthroughs by many famous historical figures have been documented over the centuries; Hippocrates, who is known as the 'father of medicine' and who was the originator of the Hippocratic Oath, was a documented practitioner of massage and physical therapy, developing their use through his teachings. Centuries later, Claudius Galenus of Pergamon (circa AD 129) further developed Hippocrates' anatomical knowledge and surgical skills, and continued the incorporation of massage in his work at the school for gladiators, to aid healing and pain control. He is thought to be the first sports therapist.

A brief history of massage

Massage is one of the oldest forms of therapy. Egyptian tomb paintings show people being massaged. In Eastern cultures, massage has been practised continually since ancient times. A Chinese book from 2700 BC, The Yellow Emperor's Classic of Internal Medicine, recommends 'breathing exercises, massage of skin and flesh, and exercises of hands and feet' as the appropriate treatment for complete paralysis, chills, and fever. In India, the traditional healing system of Ayurvedic medicine also prescribes massage for a variety of medical conditions. Physicians of ancient Greece and Rome also utilized massage as one of the primary methods to treat pain.

In Europe, doctors such as Ambroise Pare, a 16th century physician to the French court, praised massage as a treatment for various ailments. Swedish massage, the method most familiar to Westerners, was developed in the 19th century by a Swedish doctor named Per Henrik Ling. His system was based on a study of gymnastics and physiology, and on techniques borrowed from China, Egypt, Greece, and Rome.

With the foundation in 1894 of the Society of Trained Masseurs, World War I patients suffering from nerve injury or shell shock were treated with massage. By 1900, the Society had acquired the legal and public status of a professional organization, and became the Incorporated Society of Trained Masseuses. In 1920, the Society was granted a Royal Charter. It amalgamated with the Institute of Massage and Remedial Gymnastics, forming the Chartered Society of Physiotherapy. St Thomas' Hospital, London, had a department of massage until 1934. However, later breakthroughs in medical technology and pharmacology eclipsed massage as physiotherapists began increasingly to favour electrical instruments over manual methods of stimulating the tissues.

Current practice

Recently, some physical therapies used in humans have been extended to horses, yet the transfer to dogs has not been explored as fully. Therefore, little research has been conducted into muscle dysfunction in the dog. Only recently have the canine health benefits of physical therapy and massage been identified, as the popularity of sports such as 'agility', increases.

There are a few modern practitioners and teachers of the art of canine massage who have been responsible for quietly projecting the therapy to many through high-quality professional teaching. One who stands out is Patricia Whalen-Shaw, who practises and teaches in Columbus, Ohio in the USA. For many years, she has been developing the art and transferring her skills to many, not only in the USA, but in all corners of the globe. Many of the techniques shown in Chapter 6 have been adapted from, or taken from her book *Canine Massage – the Workbook*.

With canine sports growing, it is a travesty that most of the people competing with their dogs, and their trainers, are ignorant of the basic indicators of a compromised muscular system. Due to a dog's fundamental instinct to protect itself and maintain the security of the pack, it will not overtly inform us of a problem until suffering from obvious physical dysfunction. Thus we will often have to 'second guess' muscular and myofascial disorders, as the dogs, more often than not, do not show any obvious signs.

Following an injury or strain, the body will become altered by its efforts to compensate, which then means that biomechanical changes will occur. If these are allowed to remain untreated, the somatic appearance will also alter as the body adapts to the stress; sometimes pathological changes will also become evident, and can be traced back to the initial injury. Such changes usually end up being treated in isolation rather than together; sometimes, therefore, the effects are being treated instead of the cause.

The canine body, like any living body, requires balance, or homeostasis, to thrive; without this, systems can suffer. To maintain balance, all the body's systems have to work together. For example, pain in the muscular system can affect behaviour patterns (as any form of pain will affect behaviour), the digestive system (stress from pain can have an effect on digestion), and compromise the peripheral neurological system.

The repeated postural and traumatic insults of a lifetime, combined with the tensions of emotional and psychological origin, often lead to a confusing pattern of tense and contracted fibrous tissue. This may appear to the uninformed handler, for example, as an obvious lameness. This complexity of initial trauma mixed with compensatory factors can present an extremely misleading set of symptoms. It seems that, sometimes, the dog is shouting to us for an appropriate response to its crisis, and we seem to be unable to listen. Sara Wyche, in her book entitled *The Horse's Muscles in Motion* puts it very well: 'If it's the body that speaks the language, then it is the muscles that supply the words'.

Mutual grooming and touch therapy is an important component of animal pack and herd behaviour. Unlike humans, who have been conditioned to condemn touch for many reasons, many animals are aware of the power of physical manipulation to ease the soreness of muscles. This is evident when treating dogs, as they are more in touch with their bodily requirements than we are, and know what they need to ease a problem. It is, therefore, the duty of handlers to be more aware of their dog's overall health, including awareness of its muscular system. This will, then, improve the relationship between man and dog.

The purpose of this book is to provide an insight into this subject, and to demonstrate that damage of one part of the body, no matter how small, will affect the whole. Even a small repetitive injury can have the same long-term effects as a massive acute injury. Recognition of this concept can help to prevent injury, enable the handler to know when to seek professional assistance and treatment, and give the dog the opportunity to have a long and pain-free life.

Dew of the morning,
Meet the warmth of the early sun;
The colours mix as milk and honey in a bowl,
They nourish and heal;
When poured, they fall as ice,
When they touch the earth, they become water,
Cleansing where they pool.

Anon (2007)
(A handler's poem describing her experience of her dog's treatment and subsequent return to health.)

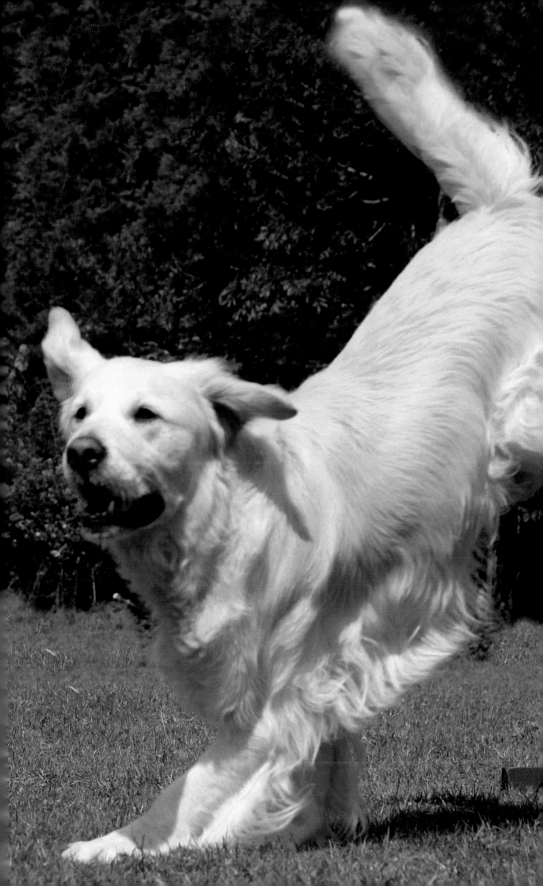

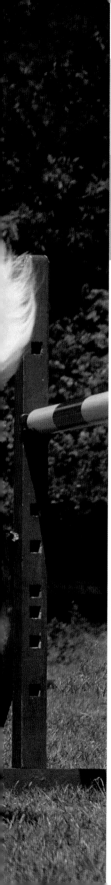

2

Anatomy and Physiology

Julia Robertson and Andy Mead

- Introduction
- Skeletal system
- Muscular system
- Fascia
- Nervous system
- Other systems
- Comparative human and canine anatomy

Introduction

A balance is required in the body on a cellular level, as it is in every part of nature. The basic requirement of every cell must be met in order for it to survive, in the same way that soil must be correctly balanced in order for a plant to grow well. If one part of a system is not working properly, it will have an effect on another part of the system and the overall performance will be compromised. This chapter will aim to show how the body works in this holistic way and how each system interacts with another. In order to understand how massage and physical therapy affect the body, it is important to understand the systems within the body, how they function, and, most importantly, how they inter-relate.

Skeletal system

The skeleton can be defined as the stiff hardened tissues that form the supporting framework of an animal's body. The skeleton is often divided into three distinct portions: the axial, the appendicular, and the visceral skeletons (2).

- The axial skeleton comprises the bones of the skull, the hyoid apparatus (larynx), the vertebral column, and the ribcage. It principally performs a protective role.
- The appendicular skeleton comprises the bones of the limbs and the bones that connect the limbs to the axial skeleton, e.g. the pelvis joining onto the sacrum.
- The visceral skeleton comprises the bones that develop in soft tissue structures. In dogs, this includes only one bone, the os penis.

It is not the intention to describe the anatomy of the canine skeleton in great detail here, as there are many other texts on the subject. Instead, an overview is presented.

Bones are a vital part of the skeletal system. They provide support and give shape to the body, as well as protecting vital organs including the heart and the brain. Above all, bones enable movement.

Bones comprise semi-rigid connective tissue and a mineral component, hydroxyapatite. The connective tissue is formed of type 1 collagen, the most common protein of connective tissue, which is made up of three polypeptide strands interlinked by hydrogen bonds into a left-handed helix. This provides an essentially brittle matrix of bone; what little capacity it has to withstand compressive and tensile forces is provided by weak hydrogen bonds between strands.

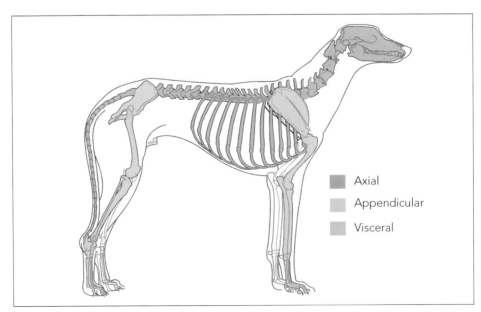

Axial
Appendicular
Visceral

2 Major divisions of the canine skeleton.

Hydroxyapatite is essentially calcium and phosphorus $(Ca_{10}[PO_4]_6[OH]_2)$ and constitutes approximately 70% of bone. It usually crystallizes in a very organized hexagonal pattern, providing rigidity to the structure of bone, as well as giving bone its smooth, white appearance. Bone also contains many different types of cells supported within the matrix, which allow the structure to grow, repair, and, perhaps more importantly, provide a scaffold for the performance of vital functions, such as red and white blood cell production.

Bone is the body's mineral store, providing a reservoir of, for example, calcium and phosphorus, which can be mobilized for the purposes of:

- Maintaining calcium homeostasis.
- Detoxifying heavy metals.
- Producing blood cells within the marrow.
- Transferring sound though the bones of the ear.

The structure of bone can be categorized into two types, compact and trabecular.

Compact bone

This forms the hard outer layer of bone, which is both smooth and well-ordered. There are minimal gaps here between collagen fibres and the mineral matrix. Compact bone is often referred to as cortical bone (3).

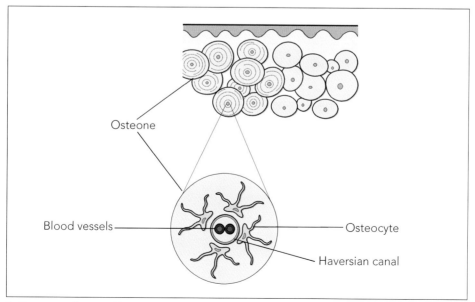

Osteone

Blood vessels

Osteocyte

Haversian canal

3 Diagram of cortical bone showing osteones and structural organization.

Trabecular bone

This forms the rather more disorganized, spongy, central portion of bone (**4, 5**). Trabecular bone reduces the total weight of a bone, as well as providing a framework for blood vessels and nerves. Without the presence of this type of bone, mammalian species would be greatly restricted in terms of size, due to the fact that greater muscle mass would be required to lift and move heavier bones. Without trabecular bone, bones of the axial skeleton would need to be as wide as they were long in order to withstand the forces put on them. Trabecular bone is often harvested surgically to aid with fracture repair.

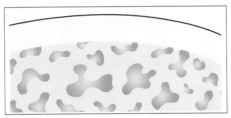

4 Trabecular bone showing disorganization of structure.

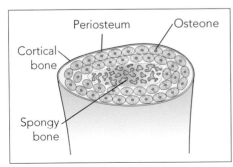

5 A section through bone showing the position of trabecular and cortical bones.

Cellular structure of bone

It is necessary to discuss in some detail the cellular structure of bone in order to understand better the process of bone development, and thereby understand how, if disturbed, these processes can lead to malformation and disease which may become significant in later life.

The main building blocks of bone at the cellular level are osteoblasts, osteocytes, and osteoclasts. These cells are present within bone throughout life. Bone is constantly being remodelled, as it is subject to ever-present stresses and strains, even at a microscopic level. Each of these constituent cells of bone has a different role in the development and maintenance of its structure, and of calcium homeostasis. All are given the prefix 'osteo', which pertains to bone.

Osteoblasts

These are bone-forming cells that produce osteoid, which is principally made up of collagen type 1. Osteoblasts have roles in the production of hormones and enzymes, most notably the enzyme alkaline phosphatase, which, among other functions, enables the mineralization of bone.

Osteocytes

Osteocytes are essentially osteoblasts which become trapped in the collagen/hydroxyapatite matrix and occupy a space within the structure called a lacuna. These cells communicate with one another through special channels and help bone to manage forces and stress, as well as playing a part in calcium metabolism. Calcium homeostasis is imperative within the mammalian body, in order to allow muscle contraction, nerve communication, and maintenance of the correct structure and rigidity of bone.

Osteoclasts

These are cells engaged in the remodelling of bone during growth or after injury.

Bone development

The process of bone development is complex, and will not be covered in great detail within this text. The embryo undergoes the process of gastrulation, which involves the early fetal cells differentiating into three distinct layers – ectoderm, mesoderm, and endoderm. It is the mesoderm layer that produces the rudimentary origins of limbs, and therefore bony tissue. The process by which bone develops from this mesoderm is known as ossification; the process is subdivided into endochondral ossification and intramembranous ossification.

Endochondral ossification

Endochondral ossification commences within the embryo and only finishes when the animal reaches maturity. Put simply, an initial scaffold of cartilage is gradually replaced with both cortical and trabecular bone tissue. Such a process accounts for the development of every long bone of the body.

The cartilage template formed within the embryo by the mesodermal cells is replaced by bone at three distinct ossification centres: the diaphysis (or middle) of each long bone, and two epiphyses, one at each end of the long bones. This process occurs from the centre outwards; long bones end up capped by cartilage which has not been ossified. This forms the articular cartilage of joints. Two discoid areas develop between the epiphyses and the diaphysis, known as growth plates or metaphyses (6). Lengthening of bone always occurs at the side of the growth plate that is closer to the epiphysis.

As previously discussed, the inner core of a long bone is spongy or less solid. It is the osteoclasts that remodel and reshape bone which results in the presence of a cavity in the centre of long bones known as the medullary cavity.

The growth plates, which remain after the differentiation of the ossification

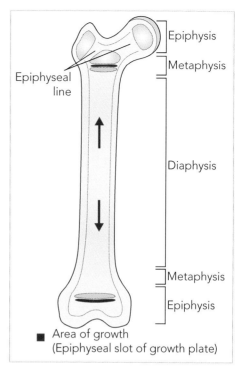

6 Endochondral ossification showing the position of diaphysis, metaphysis, and epiphysis.

centres, allow long bones to lengthen as the animal grows, long after it has left the womb. This process only stops once these growth plates close, i.e. are also ossified, a process that occurs only when an animal reaches maturity. However, these growth plates vary in the age at which they close. To the untrained eye, they can often be mistaken for fractures on radiographs.

Intramembranous ossification

This differs from endochondral ossification in that there is no cartilaginous scaffold, bone being formed directly from fibrous connective tissue. This occurs in bones such as the frontal bone, and others that form the skull.

Bone construction

The form/shape of any long bone is determined by the cortex, the outer strong layer of the bone. The cortex is arranged in a uniform manner comprising a central channel, the Haversian canal, through which blood vessels, nerves, and lymphatic vessels flow. Around this, a matrix of hydroxyapatite and collagen form concentric tubes known as lamellae. The whole system is known as an osteone (3). Within the lamellae are spaces (lacunae) which are home to the osteocytes. The whole system of lamellae, lacuna, and Haversian canals is referred to as the Haversian system, which, as previously discussed, can be densely packed, as in compact bone, or separated by much larger spaces, as in cancellous bone.

The entire surface of bone, apart from the joint capsule, is covered by a tough connective tissue, the periosteum, which has the primary role of forming attachments for muscles, tendons, and ligaments. The periosteum also has bone-forming properties which may be called upon in in the event of a fracture.

Like any other cells of the body, the cells of bone require nutrients and the removal of waste products. These are supplied and removed by an extensive skeletal blood supply which comprises 5% or more of the cardiac output. Such blood vessels, known as nutrient arteries, penetrate the cortex of bone via nutrient foramina and go on to form the tiny blood vessels of the Haversian systems.

Classification of bones

Long bones

Long bones are longer than they are wide, and consist of two epiphyses covered in articular cartilage and a diaphysis (7). These are the main bones of the limbs and their shape means that they act as levers.

Short bones

These are roughly cube shaped and consist of a core of cancellous bone covered by a layer of compact bone. Short bones are only found within the carpus and tarsus (8).

Flat bones

Flat bones consist of two plates of compact bone with a core of cancellous bone. Examples include the majority of bones in the skull and the ribs (9).

Irregular bones

These are similar to flat bones, except that they are far more complex in shape and arrangement. The vertebrae are examples of irregular bones (10).

Sesamoid bones

These are small bones buried within tendons. They reduce friction and, therefore, tendon damage, by altering the angle at which a tendon passes over a joint, allowing greater ease of movement and acting as a pivot. These specialized bones prevent tendon wear and increase leverage. The most obvious example of a sesamoid bone is the patella (11).

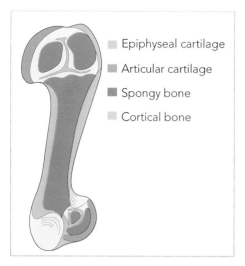

Epiphyseal cartilage

Articular cartilage

Spongy bone

Cortical bone

7 Diagram of a long bone, showing portions of spongy and cortical bone, and articular and epiphysial cartilage.

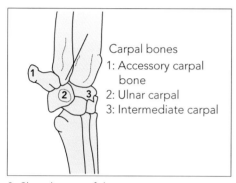

Carpal bones
1: Accessory carpal bone
2: Ulnar carpal
3: Intermediate carpal

8 Short bones of the carpus.

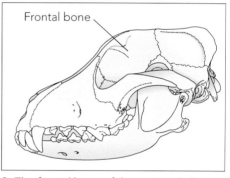

Frontal bone

9 The frontal bone of the canine skull, a flat bone.

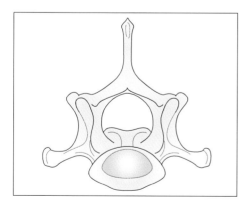

10 A lumbar vertebra, an irregular bone.

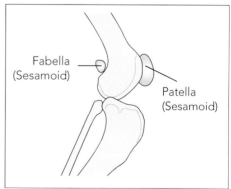

Fabella (Sesamoid)

Patella (Sesamoid)

11 Sesamoid bones such as the patella and fabella in the canine stifle joint act as pivots and allow flexion and extension.

Biomechanics of bone

When weight or stress is applied to bone, it acts like a beam of wood or steel – the force is concentrated in the outer surface, which explains why the medulla need not be solid like the cortex. Similarly, this accounts for the fact that bones are often tubular in shape. The cortex has the ability to recover from considerable deformation; however, should the osteones bend or stretch too far, stress fractures will soon appear, even if there is not enough force to break the bone in two. The majority of fractures are caused by excessive bending, stress being applied to both sides of the bone equally. However, different types of forces will affect opposite sides of the bone: one side will be affected by tensile forces pulling the cells, lamellae, collagen, and mineral components apart, and the other will be affected by compressive forces pushing structures together and crushing them (12). Generally speaking, the former are more easily dealt with by bone.

Joints

Joints are defined as the junction between two or more bones and are classified as simple or compound. Joints provide motion and flexibility to the skeleton and, perhaps most importantly, allow growth.

Different types of joints allow different amounts of movement. Indeed some joints allow no movement at all; for example, the joints of the skull; these are called synarthroses. For the purposes of physical therapy, the movable or synovial joints, by far the most common joints of the body, are the most important (13). The structure of the joint determines the type and direction of movement allowed. This provides a logical system for classification: they can be either plane, ball and socket, hinge, pivot, condylar, or saddle joints.

Movements of joints

These are divided into the following categories:

- Flexion – decreasing the inner angle between two bones, or bending the joint.
- Extension – increasing the angle, or straightening the joint.
- Abduction – pulling away from the centre or axis; for example, moving the pelvic limb laterally.
- Adduction – pulling towards the centre or axis; for example, moving the pelvic limb medially.
- Rotation – movement around an axis.
- Circumduction – circular movement of a limb.

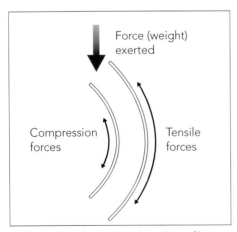

12 Forces involved in the bending of bone.

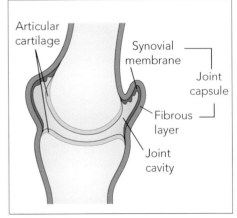

13 Synovial joint.

- Protraction – in this context, moving a limb forward.
- Retraction – pulling a limb backwards.

In the case of the elbow, a hinge joint permits flexion and extension (**14**). In the hip, a ball and socket joint allows flexion, extension, abduction, adduction, rotation, and circumduction (**15**).

Joint structure

For the purposes of this text, we shall concentrate on the structure of synovial joints. The importance of structure will become clear when discussing diseases associated with synovial joints in subsequent chapters.

In a synovial joint, the two articulating bones are divided by a fluid-filled structure, the joint cavity. The fluid (synovial fluid) is found within the joint capsule and is surrounded by a thin layer of synovial or joint fluid-producing cells, known as the synovial membrane. This is a weak structure and is often, but not always, given strength by various additional ligaments and tendons, which are designed to prevent movement in

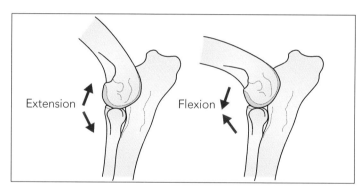

14 An elbow joint undergoing flexion and extension, medial view.

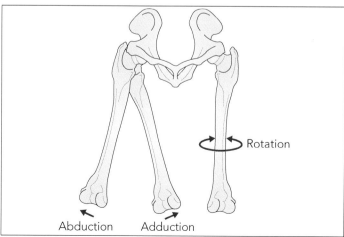

15 Dog pelvis and femora – cranial view. Rotation, adduction, and abduction of the hip joint.

certain directions and limit the amount of movement that can be achieved by a joint (16). At either end of the opposing bones and within the joint capsule is articular cartilage, a specialized form of cartilage that reduces the friction and compressive forces of locomotion. The purpose of articular cartilage is to cushion the bones and prevent wear and tear. It is smooth, elastic, and thick in the areas which require it most, i.e. the points at which the compression and friction forces are greatest.

In dogs, the articular cartilage is only 1mm thick in places; therefore, it is fragile and subject to damage from an early age. Articular cartilage has no nerve or blood supply and only receives nutrient support by diffusion from the surrounding structures, particularly the synovial fluid. Surrounding the articular cartilage within the joint capsule is the synovial fluid, which is derived from the synovial cells of the synovial membrane. The synovial membrane is a connective tissue sheet that produces the lubricant of the joint, called the glycosaminoglycans. The synovial membrane has a rich vascular supply and innervation. The fluid it produces is very viscous, its viscosity often being measured to establish the cause of various disease processes. The synovial fluid acts as a lubricant, reducing the friction between joints, and as a nutritional source for the surrounding articular cartilage.

Surrounding and encapsulating all of the above is the joint capsule, a fibrous layer. This attaches to the bone on either side of the joint and provides congruity. Proprioceptive nerves innervate these structures. The ligaments provide strength to the joints themselves.

Skeletal terminology

In order to describe the position of bony lesions accurately, it is important to use the correct anatomical terminology. The various parts of a bone's surface are called:

- Crest – a ridge of bone, e.g. the occipital crest of the skull.
- Condyle – a rounded projection of bone at a joint, e.g. the femoral condyle.
- Epicondyle – a separate, smaller prominence close to the condyle.
- Foramen – a natural opening through a bone, through which muscles, nerves, blood vessels, etc. pass, e.g. the obturator foramen of the pelvis.
- Fossa – a hollow or depression, e.g. the olecranon fossa of the elbow.
- Head – a rounded articular surface, e.g. the head of the femur.
- Tuberosity – a protuberance of a bone, e.g. the tibial tuberosity.
- Trochanter – a type of tuberosity specific to the femur and a large rough process, e.g. the greater, lesser, and third trochanters of the femur.
- Trochlea – a depression in the bone where major tendons lie forming a type of hinge, e.g. the trochlear groove of the knee joint.
- Tubercle – a small rounded process, e.g. the greater tubercle of the femur.

For the practitioner, it is important to be able to identify the palpable bony prominences of the canine, for example, the greater trochanter of the femur (17), the vertical spinous processes the ilium of the pelvis, and so on. These points of reference are far easier to palpate in the fit athletic patient and within certain breeds, for example the Greyhound. These landmarks are best described diagrammatically (18).

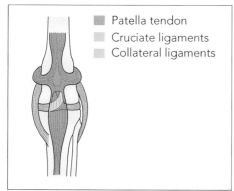

Patella tendon
Cruciate ligaments
Collateral ligaments

16 Cranial view of a simplified stifle joint, showing ligaments and tendons.

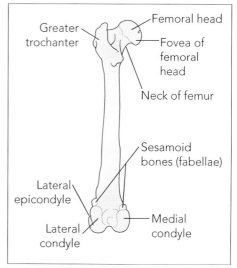

Greater trochanter
Femoral head
Fovea of femoral head
Neck of femur
Sesamoid bones (fabellae)
Lateral epicondyle
Lateral condyle
Medial condyle

17 Palpable points of the canine femur, caudal view.

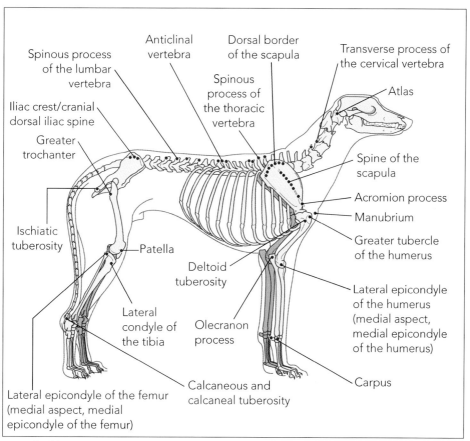

Anticlinal vertebra
Dorsal border of the scapula
Spinous process of the lumbar vertebra
Transverse process of the cervical vertebra
Spinous process of the thoracic vertebra
Atlas
Iliac crest/cranial dorsal iliac spine
Greater trochanter
Spine of the scapula
Acromion process
Manubrium
Ischiatic tuberosity
Greater tubercle of the humerus
Patella
Deltoid tuberosity
Lateral epicondyle of the humerus (medial aspect, medial epicondyle of the humerus)
Lateral condyle of the tibia
Olecranon process
Carpus
Lateral epicondyle of the femur (medial aspect, medial epicondyle of the femur)
Calcaneous and calcaneal tuberosity

18 Palpable canine bony landmarks.

Muscular system

The muscles of the body are incredibly powerful and are designed to act on the levers or joints of the body's skeletal system to initiate, drive, and sustain movement. It is important to understand how this system is designed and operates, as it directly influences the positioning and balance of the whole skeletal system. The skeletal muscular system is one of the largest systems in the dog's body and its purpose is to provide movement. There are muscles which initiate movement and others which control and stabilize. All of these must work together for the muscular system to operate effectively as a whole. Therefore, it is important to view muscles as an entity and not in isolation; they form groups that are working together, sometimes having common origins and insertions.

Muscle anatomy

There are three types of muscle; the main difference between them is the way they are innervated.

- Skeletal/striated muscle – when applying physical therapy we are primarily working with this type of muscle, which can also be referred to as 'voluntary' muscle. It is involved with movement of the body as a whole and in most dogs it accounts for about 44% of the body weight, although this rises to 57% in Greyhounds.
- Smooth/visceral muscle – this type of muscle is concerned with the control and movement of internal organs.
- Heart muscle – this is only found in the heart.

Skeletal muscles consist of densely packed bundles of elongated cells known as muscle fibres, which are held together by fibrous connective tissue. The muscle fibre, or cell, is the basic unit of contraction and it is made up of two types of protein filaments, actin and myosin (19). Thousands of these filaments group together to form myofibrils and a cluster of myofibrils form one muscle fibre. Muscle fibres are then bound together by connective tissue called endomysium to form a fascicle, which is, in turn, contained within more connective tissue, the perimysium, to form the whole muscle. Nerves and blood vessels run through and along these layers of connective tissue.

Muscles form overlapping layers in an intricate pattern over a dog's entire body. The first layers of muscles immediately under the skin are called superficial muscles, with the layers lying beneath being known as deep muscles. Muscles that span one joint are called uniaxial and those that span two joints are called biaxial. The joints they span provide movement through the articulation of the skeletal joints (see Skeletal system).

The muscles attach to bones using tendons known as insertions and origins. The origin of the muscle is generally situated closer to the body centre and the insertion, with a few exceptions, is further from the body centre. The insertion generally has the stronger attachment and, therefore, is more often the site for stress injuries.

The centre of the muscle and/or the thickest section is called the belly. Muscles and their grouping can be diverse in their anatomy; they can have more than one belly (e.g. the triceps brachii muscle, 20), or long tendinous bodies (e.g. the pectineus muscle).

The appearance of muscles varies greatly, from large muscles in the legs, which are used to perform a powerful driving movement, through to the smaller supportive muscles that provide strength and stability. Generally, it can be said that the deep muscles provide support for the

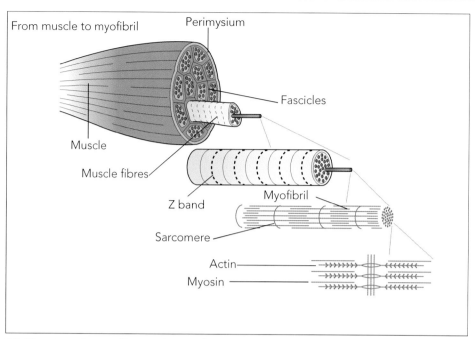

19 Structure of a myofilament in muscle.

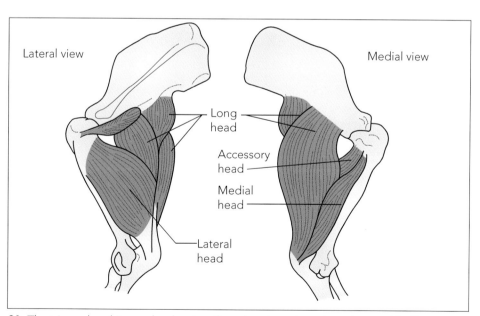

20 The triceps brachii muscle, showing three heads and one insertion, and fusiform type (medial view).

skeleton and provide strength, while the superficial muscles provide the movement. Skeletal muscles vary in shape and function; each has evolved to suit its unique purpose by its origins, insertions, and positioning:

- Fusiform ('spindle shaped') – these consist of muscle fibres which run the length of the muscle belly and converge at each end. This strap-like, round shape enables this muscle type to perform a large range of movements. This formation is generally found superficially in the larger skeletal muscles and those involved with flexion and extension of the skeletal joints to provide movement, e.g. the triceps brachii.
- Pennate ('featherlike') – these muscles tend to be flat with their fibres arranged around a central tendon. They can be unipennate (**21**), bipennate, or multipennate (**22**), depending on the arrangement around the central tendon. This formation is generally found in deep muscles that are involved with stabilizing and postural requirements for movement.
- Postural/stabilizing muscle – these support the skeleton and tend to be shorter than the 'movement' muscles. Some have several origins, and their arrangement produces the power required for maximum stability and to sustain a joint in a good position during weight transference. These muscles tend to be in various pennate fibre arrangements and are highly innervated to provide the varied and intricate movements required for joint stability. They generally have a greater proportion of slow twitch muscle fibres (see Muscle physiology).

The larger postural muscles that hold a position during a specific movement or action are called 'fixators'; an example of

these is the superficial pectoral muscle. Smaller muscles, which work to control and stabilize the overall movement in conjunction with the prime mover, are called 'synergists'; for example, the medial gluteal muscle.

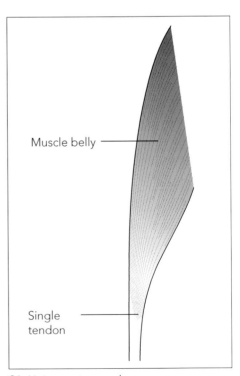

Muscle belly

Single tendon

21 Unipennate muscle.

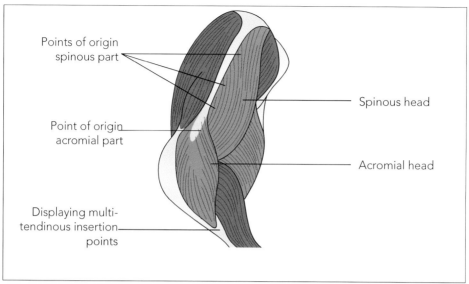

Points of origin
spinous part

Point of origin
acromial part

Spinous head

Acromial head

Displaying multi-
tendinous insertion
points

22 Multipennate deltoid muscle.

Skeletal muscles can also be classed as extrinsic or intrinsic:

- Intrinsic muscles are positioned within one area of the body, either appendicular or axial, and do not engage with the other division. For example, the deltoid muscle is intrinsic to the thoracic limb (**22**).
- Extrinsic muscles cross regions and act or move the appendicular skeleton in relation to the axial skeleton, e.g. the trapezius muscle.

The muscles that lie dorsally and ventrally to the vertebral column are divided into two groups: hypaxial and epaxial. Epaxial muscles are a complex group that is situated dorsally to the transverse processes and support, extend, and facilitate lateral flexion of the vertebral column. The hypaxial group is positioned ventrally to the transverse processes and is involved with flexion of the neck, thorax, and tail.

Muscle physiology

Voluntary muscles are stimulated to contract by electrical activity originating in nerve cells in the central nervous system (CNS). These nerves synapse with nerve cells (motor neurons) of the peripheral nervous system (PNS). The motor nerve enters the target muscle or muscles at the neuromuscular junction (NMJ) (also known as the myoneural junction), approximately two-thirds along the length of the muscle, away from its origin towards the insertion, where the nerve forms an end plate. The neural pathway carries a signal from the CNS to the muscle in the form of cellular movement of sodium and potassium ions. This signal then causes a release of calcium ions from a part of the muscle fibre called the sarcoplasmic reticulum. The muscle fibres then contract by the protein filaments (myosin and actin) sliding closer together. This shortens the overall length of the fibre, leading to a contraction of the muscle as a whole (**23**).

There are three main types of muscle fibre, differing in the types and quantities of nerves that serve the fibres. These fibre types each have different functions:

- Slow twitch type 1 – these are intended for producing lower levels of speed and power, but can operate effectively for a sustained period of time. This type of muscle fibre is dense with capillaries (bringing in

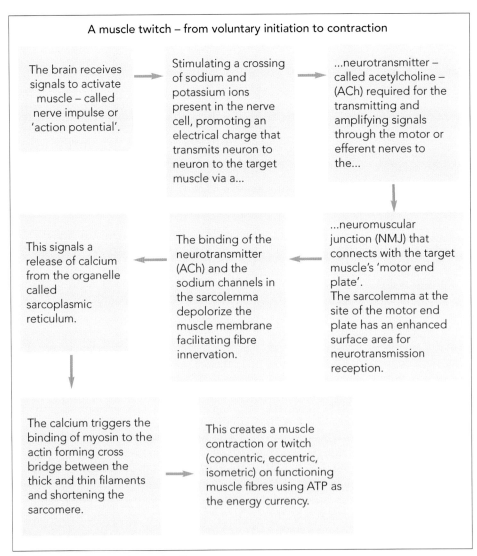

A muscle twitch – from voluntary initiation to contraction

The brain receives signals to activate muscle – called nerve impulse or 'action potential'.

Stimulating a crossing of sodium and potassium ions present in the nerve cell, promoting an electrical charge that transmits neuron to neuron to the target muscle via a...

...neurotransmitter – called acetylcholine – (ACh) required for the transmitting and amplifying signals through the motor or efferent nerves to the...

...neuromuscular junction (NMJ) that connects with the target muscle's 'motor end plate'. The sarcolemma at the site of the motor end plate has an enhanced surface area for neurotransmission reception.

The binding of the neurotransmitter (ACh) and the sodium channels in the sarcolemma depolarize the muscle membrane facilitating fibre innervation.

This signals a release of calcium from the organelle called sarcoplasmic reticulum.

The calcium triggers the binding of myosin to the actin forming cross bridge between the thick and thin filaments and shortening the sarcomere.

This creates a muscle contraction or twitch (concentric, eccentric, isometric) on functioning muscle fibres using ATP as the energy currency.

23 Algorithm for muscle contraction.

oxygen) and has many mitochondria (the 'energy factories' of a cell) and much myoglobin (the oxygen-containing component of muscle); therefore, it can sustain aerobic activity. These fibres are involved in stability and core support and contain smaller motor neurons.

- Fast twitch – there are many different divisions of this type: type 2, type 2a, type 2x, and type 2b; they are divided into groups according to their contractile speed, numbers of mito-chondria, and how much myoglobin they contain. These have higher firing frequencies than slow twitch fibres to produce the contractile speed, and with their larger fibres produce more force per motor unit.
  - Fast twitch type 2 – these fibres have the capability to contract quickly, but have poor endurance. They are involved in skeletal movement and are supplied with larger motor neurons.
  - Fast twitch type 2a – these are a small group of muscle fibres that fall between the two other categories, providing a more even combination of speed, power, and endurance.
  - Fast twitch type 2x and type 2b – these have an even higher power potential but are less resistant to fatigue and have poorer endurance than type 2.

The main difference between muscle fibres is in their innervation, or type of nerve supply. For example, the fast twitch possesses a larger motor neuron which enables it to contract faster. The proportion of fast and slow twitch fibres will be determined by the required action of the muscle, which means that a deep postural muscle will have a greater proportion of slow twitch fibres. The distribution of these different fibres is generally hereditary and cannot be altered with training. When muscles contract,

muscle fibres become shorter, fatter, and assert a force on the fascia, tendons, periosteum, and the joint. Each fibre is either fully contracted or fully relaxed. If the muscle as a whole is applying 50% effort, then half of its fibres will be contracting and the other half will be relaxed. Then, as the contracting fibres begin to experience 'fatigue', the relaxing fibres will be employed.

When a dog is fit and conditioned (see Chapter 4) for the exercise or activity in which it is participating, the time between optimum muscle function and fatigue will be greater than that of a dog that has not been prepared appropriately. For muscles to function healthily, they must be in balance, like the rest of the body, and have adequate functioning fibres, innervation, nutrition, oxygen (from the blood supply), combined with a balanced excretory process (*Table 1*). With these in balance, the chemical interplay between the CNS, PNS, and the individual muscle fibres will function effectively. When any one of these factors fails to operate, the muscle cell or fibre will be adversely affected.

Table 1 Requirements for muscle contraction (or twitch)

- Direct innervation
- Intracellular chemical balance and feedback mechanisms: sodium/potassium/calcium
- Functioning muscle fibres/cells
- Adequate glycogen store
- Adequate oxygen supply
- Adequate nutritional supply (arterial supply)
- Adequate by-product removal (venous return)

The energy provider of muscle contraction is a chemical called adenosine triphosphate (ATP) that is produced and stored in the muscle cells. The bonds between adenosine and phosphate are strong and produce much energy when the bonds are broken. Release of one phosphate results in the formation of adenosine diphosphate (ADP) plus energy. This energy source can only sustain a contraction for a matter of seconds. Creatine phosphate, which is also stored in the muscle, then provides a source of phosphate to replenish the depleted ADP, so it once again becomes ATP. However, this further replenishment of the phosphate component of ADP can only provide the energy required for muscle contraction for a further few seconds.

For more sustained and prolonged muscular contraction, glycogen derived from dietary carbohydrates and stored within the cells of the muscles, is broken down through a method involving anaerobic (oxygen-lacking) glycolysis. This process produces a source of ATP that can be used to sustain prolonged continued contractions of muscle fibres. The by-product of this continuing process is pyruvic acid, which is broken down by the oxygen supplied to the muscle fibres from arterial blood delivery and is converted into glycogen by the liver. The glycogen is then transported back to the muscle cells by the arterial blood supply. If muscle cells are in an oxygen-deficient state, pyruvic acid is metabolized to lactic acid, the presence of which can cause discomfort. It is now thought however, that rather than lactic acid being detrimental to performance, it could also be converted into a valuable source of energy by mitochondria within the muscle cells.

The neural process involved in muscular activity plays a significant role in muscle recruitment, relaxation, and, thus, the state of activity. Nerves are responsible for controlling the contraction of muscles and determining the number, sequence, and force of muscular contraction/s. The requirement of fibre recruitment and force is controlled by the afferent (sensory) nerves, running from the muscle to the CNS, and efferent (motor) nerves, running in the opposite direction. The sensory structures within the muscles (muscle spindles) lie parallel to the muscle fibres and relay constant messages back to the CNS on the length of the muscle fibre required to maintain proprioception (see Nervous system).

This system is coupled with the Golgi tendon organs (24) that are located within the tendons; these report on the tension or force being exerted through the muscle to the tendon. This information is constantly transmitted back to the brain, so there is appropriate fibre recruitment for the force required. This is important to understand when trying to enhance the range of movement during rehabilitation; it is often called 'muscle memory'.

Most movements require a force far smaller than that a muscle could potentially generate and, therefore, muscle fibre fatigue, or a reduction in muscle fibre ability to produce the required force, is unusual in normal situations. However, when muscles tire, due to a reduction or restriction of the requirements for contraction (*Table 1*), they cannot produce the required force. This is generally through a lack of conditioning (see Chapter 4), general fitness, or inappropriate muscle phasing through injury. Chemical imbalance is thought to be one area that can cause fatigue in cases of excessive training or exercise. When muscles are worked hard and trained hard, the calcium channels that supply calcium to the muscle for the myosin to bind with the actin fibres can start to leak. However, if the muscle is rested for a day or so, this internal leak can repair and normal function can resume.

A major cause of a lack of, or reduction in, muscle function is microtrauma to single muscle fibres. This can be caused through over-exertion over a period of time, repetitive strain, or minor injury. It

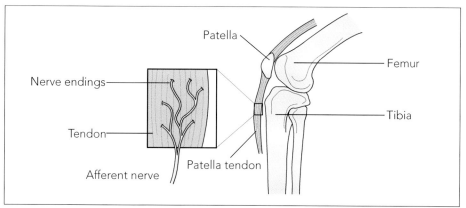

24 Diagram of a Golgi tendon organ.

can lead to post-event lameness that can either ease off with gentle exercise or, if ignored, lead to severe inflammation. This type of post-exercise 'stiffness' or lameness was once thought to be due to a build-up of lactic acid; however, it now seems that it is probably due to microtrauma within the muscle fibres.

Inability to contract a muscle is generally due to lack or reduction of excitement through the motor end plate from the serving peripheral nerve. This can be a permanent or temporary condition and can be caused by injury or disease.

Muscular coordination
In order for a muscle to contract and move a joint, the opposing muscle has to relax. Those that cause the joint to bend are called flexors, while those that straighten the joint are called extensors. To create movement, the muscles are normally paired and opposing; the one that shortens or contracts is called the prime mover or agonist, whereas the muscle that simultaneously relaxes is called the antagonist. This coordination operates through a process called reciprocal inhibition, which is a neurological reflex response. During movement, messages are transmitted through the CNS that the agonist is under tension; the reflex response to this is to inhibit the nerve input to the opposing muscle, or the antagonist, which causes it to relax, thus allowing full extension or flexion of the joint. This process helps prevent hyperextension of a joint, which can happen when there is an uneven or added force asserted through the joint.

A muscle that is tight or shortened will transmit the same message as that of one in constant contraction, therefore placing the antagonist in a state of continuing neural inhibition and causing a continued weakening. This is important to recognize when treating chronic cases involving somatic change (see Chapter 6).

Although muscle fibres can only contract and relax the muscle as a whole, a muscle can develop a force in more than one way:

- Isotonic contraction – this can be split into two categories:
  - Concentric contraction – the muscle shortens as it works, e.g. when walking or running on the flat.
  - Eccentric contraction – this is used for developing tension while lengthening, e.g. when landing after a jump, and walking or running downhill. It is used to form antagonistic tension before a movement. Every movement in the direction of gravity is controlled by eccentric contraction.
- Isometric contraction – this is where no movement is made and the muscle length remains the same when a force is applied; this can also be called static contraction, e.g. during prolonged upward head movement in obedience tests.

Muscle tone

Assessing muscular health can be extremely complex. This is due to the fact that muscles and their tone are affected by numerous circumstances. Tone (or tonus) is the partial contraction of muscle fibres to retain posture. Even when the body is asleep it retains a certain degree of tone through an autonomic neural state of balance between the motor and sensory nerves. Muscle tone is also affected by the environment and the perceived danger or excitement experienced by a dog. If the dog has no perception danger, the muscles are relaxed and the body's focus is on sustenance and rest. However, if there is any kind of positive stimulation, the muscle tone will be enhanced. This is accentuated when the dog feels his response to any impending danger is compromised, e.g. when his ability to run or fight is reduced due to muscular pain

or restriction. Thus the tone of muscles can reveal a significant amount of information about the body's state of injury or chronic dysfunction. The tone of a muscle can denote its condition (*Table 2*). Muscle can feel toned, through exercise, or tight through spasm, myopathy, or thixotropic build-up within the fibres. This final problem can be caused by chronic injury, compensatory issues, over-training, or even a lack of sufficient warming-up. Toned muscles feel soft and plump.

Table 2 The 'feel' of different muscle tones

- Healthy toned muscles – soft yet full muscle belly, good vascularization, with good potential fibre recruitment
- Hypertonic – fibres in a constant state of contraction to protect a joint/s
- Hypotonic – a lack of obvious muscle belly, a distinct deflated balloon feel. Lacking innervation through injury, lack of use, or reciprocal inhibition
- Thixotropic or fibrous – can be engorged and lacking the soft and smooth feel of a healthily toned muscle due to additional forces being constantly exerted (repetitive strain), making the differentiation of separate muscles within groups difficult
- Damaged – irregular, with a 'bubble wrap' feel

Physical disorders can result in abnormally low/poor performing (hypotonic) or high/over developed (hypertonic) muscle tone (25). Muscles can also become hypotonic or atrophied when neural impulses have been compromised either by injury or damage. In some extreme cases, an almost instant atrophy can occur; this is where the affected muscles cannot provide any tone and are unable to provide support or mobility for the surrounding joint/s. Muscle tone can also be affected by skeletal imbalances caused by injury and conformational problems. For example, if there is a dorsal tilt of the pelvis, the quadricep muscle group will be stretched, (also can be classed as hypotontic due to excessive loading) the abdominal muscles could feel flaccid, and the hamstring and adductor groups would feel tight through the shortening of the fibres, greatly reducing their usefulness (see Chapter 6), as the muscles are being recruited out of phase of their working pattern. For example, if the semimembranosus, semi-tendinosus, and biceps femoris muscles have been injured and shortened, they assert a massive force on the pelvis rather than extending the hip and providing propulsion; this then impacts on the hip flexor group, including the quadricep group, which is then put under a constant state of stretch and is therefore unable to contract or relax effectively. Conversely, if the lumbar region is tight, in some situations the hamstring group can feel hypertonic through its overuse due to the sacroiliac joint suffering reduced flexion; therefore, more drive has to come from the hamstring group.

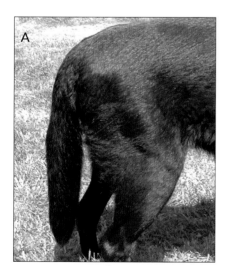
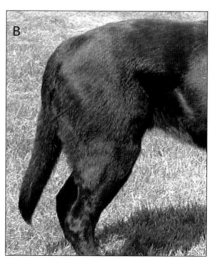

25 Comparison of muscle tone between two siblings. A: Poor muscle tone (hypotonic); the arrow is pointing to the line of the femur. Note the lack of gluteal and hamstring development and the protrusion of the femur; B: normal muscle tone; arrow pointing to biceps femoris muscle.

If a dog has a lack of mobility through illness, muscular or skeletal pain, or post-operatively, this will also cause a reduction in muscle tone. Such reduction will occur much less rapidly, and is due to a reduction of neural stimulation rather than compromised neural stimulation. Massage and passive movement (see Chapter 4) can help to retain the neural communications and improve the circulation, so as to reduce the occurrence of a chronic state of atrophy.

Knowing how muscles are phased and having good palpation skills are extremely important when assessing the condition of a muscle or muscle group (see Chapter 3). This is crucial when trying to ascertain whether a muscle is toned, thixotrophic, stretched, damaged, or in spasm. Experience enables the practitioner to learn how muscle behaves in different situations and conditions, and to diff-erentiate between a well-developed and healthy muscle and one that is unhealthy. Good palpation and assessment skills are essential for identifying the site of injury caused by a chronic insult, as surrounding muscles and fascia can provide misleading information. An accurate assessment can only be made by an experienced practitioner (see Chapter 6).

Fascia

Fascia is a fibrous connective tissue that permeates and interpenetrates tissues, enveloping the entire body. It forms a continuous network that is responsible for the supporting structure, form, and intercellular communication, all of which are needed to aid tissue repair. Fascia is uninterrupted, and because it extends through muscle, bones, nerves, and blood vessels, it forms an extremely effective communication matrix spanning the whole body. It also assists tissue repair through the complex intercellular com-munication network. Through its physical construction and connective properties, it also supports and aids protection for internal organs. Due to these continuous and contiguous properties, it enables us to view the body as a system of continuous networks of tissues, and not merely an assembly of separate parts.

In veterinary research, fascial connec-tions are still fairly unexplored. Even within human scientific research, the study of fascia as an organ of support has been largely neglected, and its role in musculoskeletal function and dysfunction has received relatively little attention. This may be due to fascia's far-reaching effects, which make it difficult to study; it cannot be easily divided into units and subunits.

Even within the fields of dissection and surgery, fascia has always been viewed as obscuring the anatomical structures of interest, such as muscles, nerves, and blood vessels. However, we must remember that the tissue removed is responsible for the support, connection, separation, and, most importantly, the interdependence of the structures being investigated (26). We can only look to human research to see how bodies are connected by these fascial chains; this can help us to answer many questions when treating dogs. Thus, it is necessary to think of fascia as a complete supportive system. Tracing and linking the muscles by following the chain of these fascial connections to an original point of injury is an important skill for a practitioner.

Anatomy of fascia

The two main areas of fascia that are relevant are superficial and deep:

- Superficial fascia – lies just below the skin in most of the body.
  The superficial fascia of the trunk corresponds to the subcutis, envelopes the cutaneous muscles, and lies directly under the skin of most regions of the body. It contains mainly areolar and adipose connective tissue, and therefore can support and store fat, providing insulation and protection. It also supports blood, lymph, and nerve vessels.

- Deep fascia – encloses individual muscles. It forms loose connections with adjacent muscles, forms attachments to bone, directs muscle contraction, and supports and secures internal organs. It is a dense fibrous connective tissue that permeates muscles, and separates groups. It provides physical connection and neural communication between the muscles through fascial linking of tendons and fascial attachments called aponeuroses. These are wide fibrous, tendon-like structures that increase the area of muscle attachment and the anchorage of muscle to bone. These fascial attachments form uninterrupted chains supporting much of the body. This continuous network has an active role in cellular innervation, which regulates activity. It is also a matrix for these highly organized structures, including pathways for nerves, capillaries, and lymphatic vessels that serve the muscle.

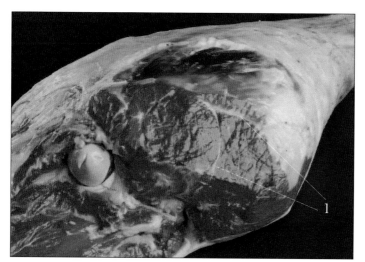

26 Fascial bands separating the hamstring group of muscles in a leg of lamb. 1: Fascial bands.

Thus, the practitioner must not view muscular functions individually, but think more of interrelations and connections between one muscle and another, and the fascial relationship between them. This continuous structure, when damaged, can cause either far-reaching or local problems, forming adhesions to adjacent structures. When damaged, fascia can rupture, tear, or become inflamed and painful. It has a smaller blood supply than many tissues, which can lead to poor healing.

CASE STUDY 1

Tia, an extremely active Border Collie that competed at a high level in agility, suffered an accident that led to pelvic limb ataxia during exercise. Her handler took her to her veterinary surgeon, but by this time she was regaining limited movement of her pelvic limbs. She was then referred for a magnetic resonance imaging (MRI) scan, but it gave no explanation for her condition. Therefore, no solution could be offered. Tia was then sent for myotherapy treatment 4 weeks post-accident. She presented as a dog that had the look of a jack-knifing lorry: her front end was moving forwards and her back end was following its own disunited course. Following palpation by the Galen myotherapist, a tear was found within the fascial connection of the left side of m. latissimus dorsi; the tear was about 1.5 inches (3.5 cm) wide and presented like a circular indent with raised edges. Could this have been the reason for the temporary loss of use of the limbs? More importantly, could this be the reason for her lack of pelvic stability (27)? The m. latissimus dorsi joins the thoracic limb to the pelvis through the thoracolumbar fascial plane, and therefore has a stabilizing role.

After 5 months, Tia is following a course of rehabilitation exercises (see Chapter 5) and regular treatment from a myotherapist; the scar tissue is being managed and her core stability is being enhanced. Her quality of life is very good, but she obviously misses her agility classes.

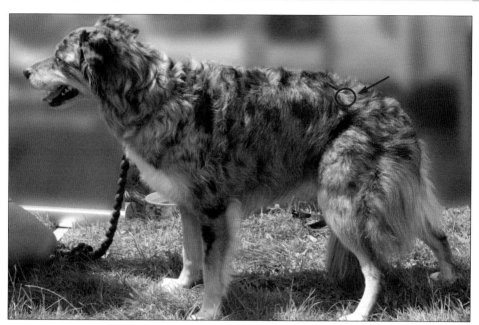

27 Tia, showing her typical stance, compensating for a lack of structural stability. The arrow indicates the position of the fascial tear.

Fascia and muscle

The role of fascia in relation to muscle tissue is that of constraint, containment, and connection, to allow the energy produced from the fibres to remain concentrated and focused or, conversely, distributed to surrounding tissues as required by biomechanics. This avoids any power dissipation during activity, through tensile strength and elasticity of the outer fascial sheath. This keeps the muscle in its correct position, whether in contraction or not, and sustains the loose fascial connection with adjacent muscles to maintain alignment and orientation in both situations. Any form of fascial tear will compromise the muscles' or muscle group's integrity (see Case study 1).

How do the combinations of muscles and fascial planes impact on the biomechanics of the dog? This can be answered by looking at anatomical trains. Within the human form, anatomical trains, or the myofascial planes, are well documented; considering the similarity of our musculoskeletal system to that of the dog, we can view the dog in the same way. Thus, we can achieve a much more three-dimensional feel for body patterns, compensatory effects, and strain distributions; these would otherwise be treated in isolation.

'The anatomy train is a line of tensional pull, not compressional push – therefore, it must, like any functioning tensile apparatus, follow the most straight lines, both in direction and depth'.

Tom Myers

Dissection has demonstrated human anatomy trains (**28**); five of the same trains have been postulated to occur in the dog through observation, and appropriate treatment programmes (**29**). These areas are worthy of note and can challenge traditional methods of assessment.

Myofascial stress

The stresses of movement have a piezo-electric effect on the surrounding molecules, which causes the bonds between them to be stretched. This slight electrical flow is communicated and interpreted by the cells in close proximity, causing them to respond and reorganize the intercellular elements in the area. This includes bone formation and density due to exercise, and the stress lines in each individual (see Skeletal system). This can be affected by the stresses caused through

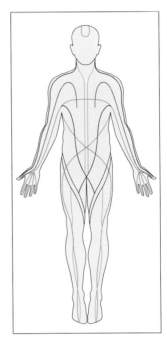

28 Based on Human Anatomy Trains™. (Courtesy of Tom Myers.)

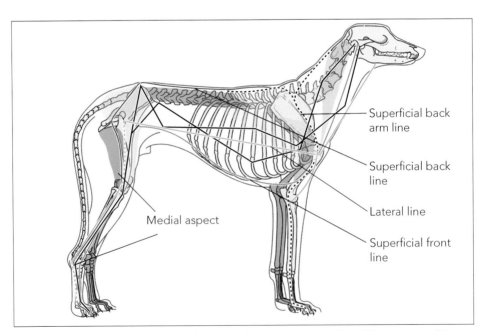

Superficial back arm line

Superficial back line

Lateral line

Superficial front line

Medial aspect

29 Postulated canine fascial trains (based on human Anatomy Trains™, courtesy of Tom Myers). Not all the trains are featured; all four legs should have four lines each: cranial and caudal for mobilization and lateral and medial for stabilization.

injury, overuse (especially in puppyhood), or chronic repetitive strain. Osteoblasts lay down new bone anywhere within the periosteum, and osteoclasts are controlled neurologically only to clear new bone that is not piezo-electrically charged. Therefore, over time the stresses caused through a myofascial–skeletal dissonance could have a long-term effect over the stress distribution of bones and, therefore, over joints and their application.

While not overemphasizing their importance in treatment considerations, these possible canine anatomical maps may prove to be the 'missing link' in a nonreceptive case of persistent intermittent lameness. In many cases, the release of fascial tension can prove to be a highly successful treatment.

Within the dog's skin, fascial changes can be clearly felt and assessed. The degree of change can be calculated (especially in a young dog) by the degree of elasticity displayed. When a dog is older (>10 years), the collagen is less elastic; however, there should still be a visible pliability in the skin and in surrounding tissues. If the superficial fascia is not demonstrating pliability, the dog will be displaying symptoms of somatic dysfunction, whatever its age.

Fascia and posture
There are certain specialized forms of deep fascia that stabilize and maintain a dog's posture during movement (30). They form part of the body's fascial network (29).

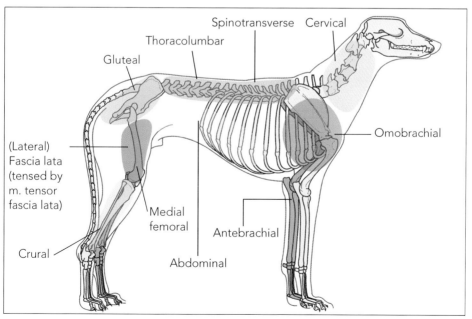

30 Canine deep fascia involved in posture.

CASE STUDY 2

Digby, an agility dog damaged the left thoracic palmar surface of his leg on glass, and was left 9/10 lame on this leg. Being a lively dog, this was not going to hold him back, despite being cage rested. When he did have exercise, the activity levels were high. When the leg healed, he was left with a chronic stiffness within the pelvic region. This was not unexpected, due to the compensatory issues he had received, but the unusual factor was that the main problem arose from the same side and not, as is the usual case, from the opposite side to the original injury (compensatory issues tend to cross diagonally or criss-cross the body). Again, this can occur, but the significance was that, when the neck was treated, there was an obvious and major skin reflex that imitated the fascial superficial front line. It travelled at a mid-point in a transverse direction across the ribs where it continued from the iliac crest in a ventral direction to his stifle. After this treatment, all stiffness eased and he resumed his agility career.

CASE STUDY 3

Jess, a 12-year-old Beagle was becoming stiffer (over the whole body) and grumpier with every week that passed. She had been treated in the same way as other successful cases by targeting hypertonic muscles, but to no avail and remained chronically lame. As a last resort the practitioner applied some thorough and very painful skin-rolling. All the skin across the thoracic and pelvic region was adhered, so this process was more than a little uncomfortable; however, a few days later, Jess was a changed dog and resumed being her affectionate self. The stiffness eased to such a point that she could resume walks and did not require any further treatment.

Consider the gravitational and mobility stresses that a dog puts its body through. The twisting, turning, and pivoting by far exceeds most human capability and sustainability (see Chapter 3). This has always been a phenomenon the author has found hard to understand when treating different dogs for various injuries. It can help to consider the skeleton, with the only soft tissue in place being the ligaments; this is anything but a stable structure against the aforementioned forces. But, then add the muscles, which can be considered to be the struts or cables that connect this bridge-like structure, and then think of a dog performing leaping and twisting movement (31).

The ligaments, cartilage, and bursae of a joint form a very resilient compression and resistance mechanism, but there are also forces in a lateral/medial direction to contend with. The 'myofascial net', in its tensional state, resists this lateral movement and pulls inwardly towards the centre, providing both the required stability and practical mobility.

This is just the beginning of our discovery of the amazing qualities and importance of fascia as a connective tissue, and I hope that this section has in some way begun to explain and demonstrate the qualities of connective tissue and how it should be viewed when assessing a dog's injury pathway.

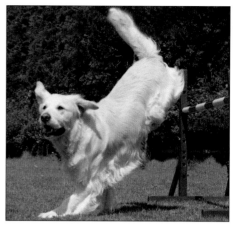

31 The combined concussional and twisting effect of a dog jumping.

Nervous system

The nervous system is the control centre of the body. It processes hundreds of thousands of pieces of information every second in order to respond to external stimuli, and thus ensure the appropriate response to a situation or environment. Neurology/neuroanatomy is a discipline often feared and ignored, due to the complicated structure of the nervous system, the myriad of tracts, nerves, divisions, and their varying terminologies. An in-depth knowledge of spinal tracts and microscopic neuroanatomy is commendable, but not essential, here. Basic terminology is, however, required and will be covered in some detail by this text.

The nervous system consists of the brain, the spinal cord, and the myriad of peripheral nerves that branch from these structures, transmitting impulses to the far reaches of the body. The brain and spinal cord comprise the CNS (**32**), and the peripheral nerves make up the PNS (**33**).

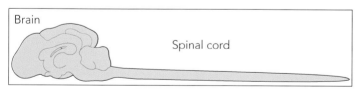

Brain

Spinal cord

32 Schematic diagram of the central nervous system.

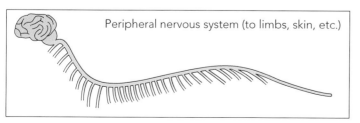

Peripheral nervous system (to limbs, skin, etc.)

33 Schematic diagram of the peripheral nervous system.

Imagine that the CNS is similar to a computer, sending, storing, and evaluating information. The PNS is represented by everything connected to the computer, e.g. the mouse, keyboard, and so on. Each is useless without the other; the CNS cannot transmit impulses to the periphery of the body without the PNS, and the PNS has no purpose without the CNS sending it information. Indeed, the nervous system consists of super-fast communication channels that allow stimuli to be detected and an appropriate response to be implemented rapidly. Furthermore, just as a computer hard drive retains photographs or documents, the brain stores this information so that previous experiences can be drawn upon and learned from. This enables both animals and humans to be better prepared to deal with similar events in the future.

A further distinction is made according to the type of nerve impulse carried by the nerve:

- Sensory (afferent) nerves – carry information regarding the environment, e.g. position or temperature. Such information is relayed to the CNS to process. The information ascends from the peripheral nerves via tracts in the spinal cord to the brain.
- Motor (efferent) nerves – carry information from the brain and spinal cord to the periphery in order to adjust to the information provided by sensory nerves, adapt to surroundings, and react to various stimuli. Efferent nerves travel away from the CNS. Put simply, the motor system instructs and allows muscle to contract and relax.

The motor system is then further divided into the upper motor neuron (UMN) and lower motor neuron (LMN) systems, depending on where these motor neurons send information from and to (34). The UMN system consists of motor nerves going from the brain to the spinal cord, which then synapse with the LMN, connecting muscles, glands and the rest of the periphery of the body and effect (cause) a response. Returning to the analogy of the computer, should the LMN (e.g. the keyboard), become detached, there will be no pathway to pass sensory information back to the CNS. Pathology that affects the LMN can therefore be just as devastating as damage to the CNS. In fact, damage to the LMN will often result in catastrophic and rapid muscle atrophy, which may well lead to inability to walk or weightbear.

A distinction is also made between the portions of the nervous system which allow voluntary movement and interaction with the environment (the somatic nervous system) and those that carry involuntary information, about which we have little conscious control, the autonomic nervous system (ANS). The ANS which is further divided into the parasympathetic and sympathetic nervous systems. Sympathetic fibres are more numerous; every spinal nerve and most cranial nerves carry these fibres. The parasympathetic system is restricted to a few cranial nerves, such as the vagus nerve (cranial nerve X), which carries information to the thoracic and abdominal region, and, as the pelvic nerves, supplies the bladder and rectum.

The fundamental difference between these two nervous systems is in their functions: the parasympathetic promotes a state of rest, increasing secretion of enzymes for digestion, slowing the heart rate, and slowing peristalsis of the gut. Conversely, the sympathetic system causes an active state, initiating a 'fight or flight' response in adverse situations. It increases blood flow to the muscles and increases the heart rate.

Anatomy of the nervous system

Neurons (nerve cells)

Neurons consist of a cell body, nucleus, and two types of nerve process, called

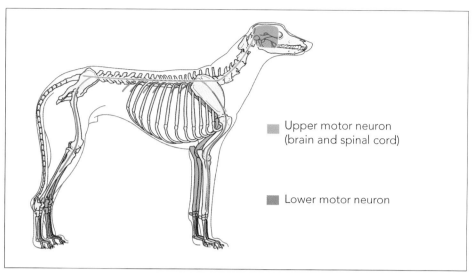

34 Lower and upper motor neuron systems.

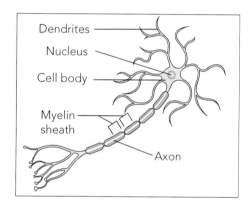

35 Schematic diagram of a neuron.

axons and dendrites (**35**). Axons carry information away from the cell body. The dendrites, which are more numerous, receive information from adjacent neurons and transmit it to the cell body in order to cause a response. The multitude of dendrites allows communication between several nerve cells, and ensures that any significant stimuli can be accurately relayed. Neurons have been considered unable to divide, so once they are damaged, function is lost.

Neuroglial cells

These are more abundant than nerve cells; they are binding cells, and also provide nutrients to neurons, especially during the process of repair.

Nerve cell communication

Communication between adjacent nerve cells and between nerve cell and target organ is made possible by way of a structure known as a synapse (36). The gap between the cell receiving information and the cell imparting it is bridged by neurotransmitters, namely acetylcholine, noradrenaline, and adrenaline. These substances bind to receptors and stimulate an impulse in the postsynaptic cell via the release of calcium. Synapses also allow this information to be passed to muscle cells via a specialized type of synapse, known as the neuromuscular junction (see Muscular system).

Nerve impulses are an 'all or nothing' phenomenon; in other words, a full impulse is either created, or not at all. Importantly, however, the degree of the response can be finely tuned by concentrating the nerve impulses to particular areas, or by reducing the number of impulses sent. It is also important to realize that not all nerve impulses are excitatory; in fact, the majority are inhibitory, ensuring that the neurological response to situations is finely tuned. The nervous system is the control centre of the body. It processes hundreds of thousands of pieces of information every second in order to respond to external stimuli, and thus ensures the appropriate response to a situation or environment.

CNS

The CNS consists of the brain and the spinal cord. The brain is the portion of the CNS contained within the skull. It has three main parts: the cerebrum, cerebellum, and the brainstem (37). Each part has a fundamental function:

- The cerebrum – performs the highest function: it is the 'thinking' portion of the brain in the human, interpreting messages and computing the appropriate response. Voluntary movement is controlled by the cerebrum.
- The cerebellum – is positioned behind the cerebral cortex. Its job is to coordinate motor reflexes and responses. It computes information that allows fine tuning of movement and balance. It also aids in proprioception.

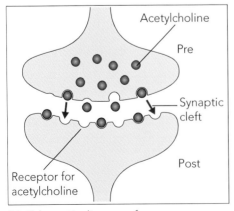

36 Schematic diagram of a synapse.

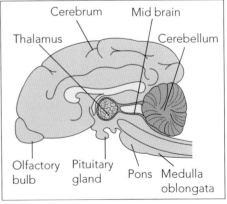

37 Schematic diagram of the brain.

- The brainstem – is further divided into the diencephalon, the mesencephalon, the pons, and the medulla oblongata. These portions contain centres to detect smell, sight, and taste, release hormones, and bridge the gap between the nervous and endocrine systems. For example, the hypothalamus controls the autonomic nervous system, regulating heart rate, temperature, water retention by the kidney, and so on.

The CNS continues from the brain in a long column, the spinal cord, within the protective bony structure known as the vertebral canal. It extends to the lumbosacral region. The vertebral column is divided into the cervical, thoracic, lumbar, and sacral regions. The number of vertebrae within each region varies by species; the dog has seven cervical, 13 thoracic, and seven lumbar vertebrae (**38**). From a spinal cord segment, a pair of spinal nerves originates

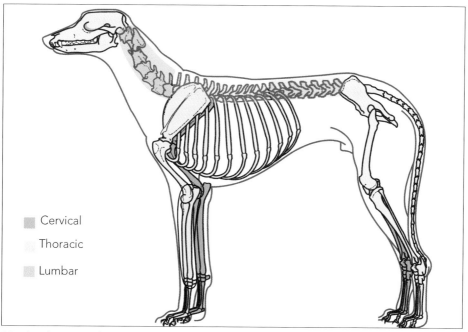

Cervical

Thoracic

Lumbar

38 The divisions of the spine in the dog.

and innervates structures within the vicinity; for example, the cervical spine serves the forelimbs, the lumbar spine serves the pelvic limbs; one nerve travels left, the other right (**39**). The spinal nerve is itself divided into the dorsal and ventral roots: the dorsal root carries sensory fibres toward the spinal cord and the ventral root carries motor fibres away.

A spinal plexus is a network of spinal nerves. For example, the brachial plexus supplies the forearm and contains, among others, the radial and ulna nerves. If a plexus is damaged by trauma or neoplasia, the results can be catastrophic as many nerves will be affected.

PNS

The PNS consists of the myriad of peripheral nerves that join the CNS to all of the body's structures, such as muscles, glands, and the vital organs (see **33**).

Cranial nerves

Twelve cranial nerves exit the brain to supply nearby peripheral structures. These can receive sensory impulses and supply motor impulses simultaneously. They form part of the PNS and are named according to their function. All, save the optic and olfactory cranial nerves, exit from the brainstem, and they are all given a roman numeral to indicate the order in which they exit, from cranial to caudal:
I – Olfactory (smell).
II – Optic (sight).
III – Oculomotor (eye movement).
IV – Trochlear (fine movement of eye).
V – Trigeminal (sensory to the forehead, nasal cavity, and cornea; motor to mandible, chewing).
VI – Abducens (motor to eye).
VII – Facial (facial expression, taste, salivation, and tear production).
VIII – Vestibulotrochlear (hearing and balance).
IX – Glossopharyngeal (taste, swallowing, salivation).
X – Vagus (swallowing, vocalization;

parasympathetic fibres to heart, lungs, liver, and so on, slows heart rate and allows digestion).
XI – Accessory (movement of the neck, swallowing, vocalization).
XII – Hypoglossal (movement of the tongue, swallowing).

Reflex arcs

Reflexes are the body's immediate responses to stimuli which occur unconsciously; they are involuntary and immediate. A reflex is 'built in' to the nervous system and does not require thought. The distance between sensor and effector is as short as possible, in order to reduce the time taken for the impulse to travel. Fundamentally, these are local responses to local stimuli. A reflex arc requires three components: a sensory nerve to 'convey' the stimulus (carrying information from a specialized receptor to detect, for instance, heat, cold, moisture, pain), an interneuron to communicate with it, and a motor neuron to carry information regarding the response (**40**). For example, should sensory neurons detect excessive heat near a finger, the correct response would be to withdraw the finger from the source of the heat. Sensory information about an unpleasant stimulus, such as a toe pinch, will thus travel to the CNS of an animal; as a result, not only might it attempt to remove the toe from the noxious (unpleasant) stimulus (a reflex response), but it may also be tempted to bite (a conscious decision)! Reflexes can be tested by a veterinary surgeon to examine the state of the nervous system when assessing the cause of lameness. The presence or absence of such reflexes is indicative of the position of damage to the nervous system.

Sensory receptors

The body is able to identify, measure, and respond to various stimuli which affect the internal and external environments.

Changes in the internal and external environment of the body must be monitored closely so that the appropriate and justifiable action may be taken. These responses may be required to protect the body; for example, removing a limb from a source of intense heat or cold, of which we are aware, to those 'internal events' of which we are not, such as changes in blood pressure or joint position (proprioception).

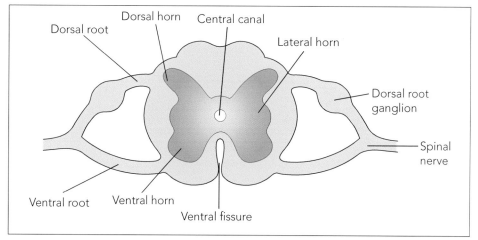

39 A spinal cord segment.

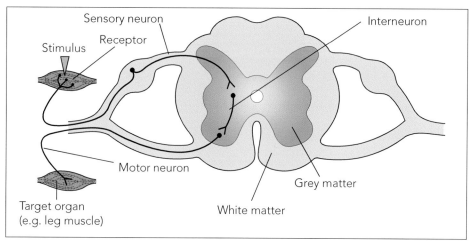

40 Schematic diagram of a reflex arc.

The types of stimuli which are detected by sensory receptors within skin, muscle, and tendons are: pain (**41**), temperature, touch (pressure, vibration, and texture), and proprioceptive stimuli. Proprioception appears to be the 'odd one out' in this group; we are aware of many other stimuli, but not of the constant subtle movements of muscle tendons and joints going on 'behind the scenes' that allow vertebrates to stand or move (**42**).

In order to detect these stimuli, specialist receptors are required, designed to respond only to a single type of stimulus. These receptors transmit information in order to trigger reflexes or responses from higher levels within the CNS. These cells are able to transmit the magnitude of the stimulus applied; a larger stimulus excites more of these higher areas in the CNS. Thus, these cells act as transducers, converting the stimuli to an 'action potential', an electrical signal that is transmitted to the CNS, where it can be interpreted.

The site of the stimulus must also be conveyed. Each receptor has a 'receptive field', a region of sensitivity within which a stimulus will activate the receptor and trigger a response. The impulse then travels via a nervous pathway to reach the sensory cortex of the brain at a specific location related to the position of the stimulus.

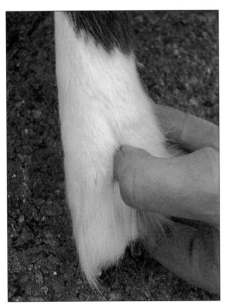

41 Reflex response to a painful stimulus. The limb will be withdrawn.

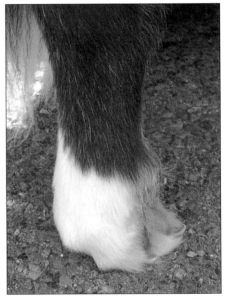

42 Proprioceptive deficits are tested by turning the foot over. A normal animal should immediately replace the foot in a normal position.

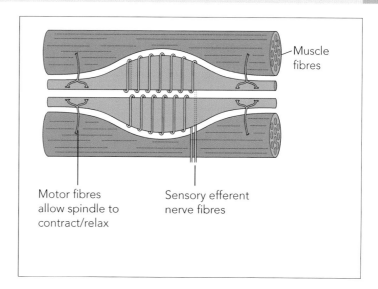

Muscle fibres

Motor fibres allow spindle to contract/relax

Sensory efferent nerve fibres

43 Schematic diagram of a muscle spindle.

The sensations of touch, pressure, and vibration are transmitted through four different receptors within the skin: Meissner's corpuscles, found in nonhairy skin such as the foot pads; Pacinian corpuscles, found within facial tissues and which are stimulated by rapid movement; Merkel's discs, cells that respond to the vertical displacement of skin; and Ruffini endings, which detect vertical and lateral movement of skin and deep fibrous tissue.

The sense of position relies upon further sensory receptors found in muscles, tendons, and on joint surfaces. In muscle, they take one of two forms, either muscle spindles or Golgi tendon organs (GTOs). Each has a distinct role: the muscle spindle gives sensory information pertaining to stretch, and the GTO relays information about the tension within tendons.

Golgi tendon organ
When a muscle is relaxed, the collagen bundles of the tendon have no tension. As soon as a tensional force is applied, the nerve endings of the GTO are laterally compressed, giving rise to an action potential and propagating a nerve impulse. The GTO cannot differentiate between passive and active contraction, and are less sensitive than muscle spindles. The stretching of collagen fibres within the GTO causes an action potential of a magnitude relative to the stretch applied, to be transmitted from the muscle to the CNS for interpretation (see **24**).

Muscle spindle
Muscle spindles are located within a capsule deep within and parallel to muscle bellies. They contain intrafusal muscle fibres, which are specialist muscle fibres innervated by both sensory and motor nerve fibres, in a spiral configuration (**43**). These intrafusal fibres are able to stretch and contract just like those of normal muscle, so the receptors are able to respond to forces of contraction and relaxation. This is enhanced by motor

efferent nerve fibres, nerve fibres that carry impulses from the spinal cord. If this were not the case, should surrounding muscle fibres contract, the muscle spindle would become unloaded, be unable to contract in sympathy, and therefore impulses generated by the stretching of the spindles would cease. Sensory information would subsequently only be generated once the muscle was stretched almost to capacity once more.

In addition, mechanoreceptors, called Ruffini endings, are present within every joint, their role being to detect compressive forces. These are similar to GTOS and are found within ligaments surrounding the joint. They signal the position of a joint, as well as its velocity and direction of movement.

Sensory information from these receptors is transmitted via one of two special pathways. In order to maintain balance, signals are sent constantly via these pathways to alter muscle tone. Indeed, we or our canine friends would fall victim to gravity without this input from sensory receptors in skin, muscle, and joints. Usually, this is combined with information from the visual cortex clarifying one's position in space and a sense of 'acceleration', transmitted by the vestibular apparatus in the inner ear.

Cerebellum

It is the job of the cerebellum to interpret the huge volumes of sensory information received from the peripheral receptors, the vestibular apparatus, and the visual cortex, in order to coordinate a response by efferent impulses transmitted from the cerebral cortex to the muscles. A lesion within the cerebellum will not cause paralysis, but it will lead to tremors or poorly controlled, exaggerated movements. The cerebellum can differentiate signals from different limbs. The planning of the next movement, the alteration of contraction of certain muscles, and the flexion or extension of joints is all undertaken by the cerebellum. This can be a likened to a chess game, but one where each move is played out in a split second.

Nerve damage

Damage to either part of the nervous system will result in characteristic clinical signs. A veterinary surgeon will observe and test for various reflexes, which will be discussed in further detail later in the chapter. Information gleaned from various reflex tests, together with an animal's demeanour, mental state, and clinical history aid in the diagnostic process and give prognostic indications.

Usually, CNS damage cannot be repaired. LMNs leave the spinal cord to innervate muscles. Damage to these nerves results in flaccid paralysis/paresis. Muscle tone is either absent or reduced. Spinal reflexes are also therefore reduced. As previously mentioned, muscles atrophy very quickly with LMN damage.

Damage to UMNs results in an inability to initiate voluntary movement; however, the reflexes are usually intact, e.g. if pinched on the toe the dog can flex its limb, often in an exaggerated manner, but it cannot walk or stand. Inhibition of LMNs is also reduced, meaning muscle tone is often normal to increased. Atrophy is slow, and, therefore, it is often more difficult to spot than LMN damage. If the UMN system is damaged in the region between the sixth cervical vertebra and the second thoracic vertebrae or between the fourth lumbar vertebra to the second sacral vertebrae, different symptoms are apparant. Between these points, peripheral nerves (LMNs) leave the spinal cord (UMNs) to innervate the thoracic and pelvic limbs respectively. In such cases, reflexes will be absent; this aids in the diagnosis of UMN and LMN damage.

Brain lesions vary in their effects; this depends on the area that is damaged:

- Lesions of the forebrain result in behavioural modification, blindness, and seizures.
- Lesions of the brainstem result in weakness, ataxia, and, potentially, paralysis.
- Lesions within the cerebellum result in poor balance, intention tremors, and often there is a wide-based stance.
- Damage to the spinal cord may cause paralysis, depending on the position of the lesion.

The very last sensation to be lost after spinal cord trauma is the deep pain response. This is normally tested by squeezing the web between the toes with forceps, causing withdrawal of the limb in the normal dog. This is often used as a prognostic indicator post-trauma. In dogs, loss of deep pain is usually indicative of a poorer outcome than if it were still present, i.e. there will be reduced likelihood of a return to normal function.

Other systems

Skin

The skin, or common integument, is said to be the body's largest and most sensory organ. It covers the entire outer surface of the dog, except for various natural openings, e.g. the mouth and anus. The integument also includes the hair, footpads, and claws. The functions of the skin go further than just supporting the coat; it also forms a physical protection from bacteria, water, chemicals, and, in pigmented skin, ultraviolet radiation. It produces various secretions from a variety of glands. One is sebum, secreted by sebaceous glands; this can be used as an antiseptic against microorganisms. It can also have a distinct odour which can indicate imbalances within a dog.

The skin consists of two layers:

- The epidermis, which is the surface layer, consisting of stratified squamous cells.
- The dermis, which is the deeper layer; its structure is more complex: it is a connective tissue layer, consisting of dense fibrous, collagenous tissue. The dermis rests on an underlying layer of connective tissue called the subcutaneous layer or subcutis. This, along with the fatty layer below, called the panniculus adiposus, forms the superficial fascia; this gives skin its flexibility (see Fascia). Both layers support blood and lymphatic vessels, nerves, and adipose tissue (**44 overleaf**).

The skin also produces sweat from specialized sweat glands in the footpads. It can also produce vitamin D from a component in the sebum that, when activated by the kidneys, can increase the uptake and metabolism of dietary calcium. The skin is also an efficient energy storage organ: adipose tissue, or subcutaneous fat, can act as an energy store or thermal insulating layer, depending on the needs of the dog. Even though sweat is not the primary method of cooling in the dog, the skin acts as a highly effective thermoregulatory instrument by either affecting vaso-constriction or dilation, diverting blood away to insulate against the cold, or dilation to assist core heat removal. This works in conjunction with the dog's panting, which is the major method of heat removal.

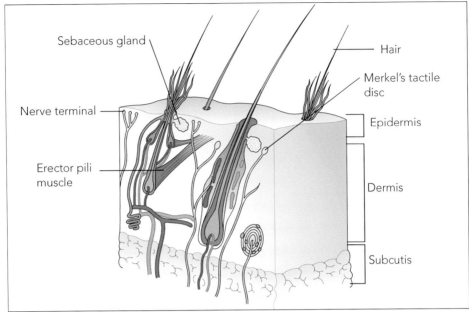

Sebaceous gland

Hair

Merkel's tactile disc

Nerve terminal

Epidermis

Erector pili muscle

Dermis

Subcutis

44 Cross-section of canine skin.

The skin is highly innervated, the function of which is to constantly maintain contact with the outside world, and then communicate this information back to the internal body systems so they can react appropriately to maintain homeostasis. It contains both sensory and motor nerves and records pressure, tension, pain, itching, vibration, stretching, heat, and cold. The most common neural receptors are Merkel's tactile discs; these detect touch and vertical displacement of skin. There are others that serve as receptors to pain; these penetrate the epidermis at multiple sites. There are also other receptors that detect heat and cold (thermoreceptors) and stretching (mechanoreceptors) (see Nervous system).

The cooling mechanism must be respected if a dog becomes excessively hot – the skin must not be covered by anything, especially anything cold, as this will reverse the body's cooling process and cause vasoconstriction and drive the escaping heat back to the core of the dog. The physical therapist operates with this complex and far-reaching network; via these neural receptors the masseur can command a degree of cellular control over the dog. The therapist must, therefore, clearly understand the treatment methodology they are employing.

The feel of the skin is an important assessment tool for the practitioner. It should be free and loose enough to 'make another dog' in most cases, but this depends on the age and breed. Tight areas or a cutaneous reflex will be indicated by a quiver, either locally or spreading distally, indicating that there could be a minor neural and/or fascial problem (see Chapter 6).

Cardiovascular system

The cardiovascular system contains the heart and blood vessels (arteries and veins). These divide into smaller vessels called arterioles and venules, respectively, which then divide again into a system of capillaries. The heart acts as a pump, transporting oxygenated arterial blood through the body, and deoxygenated blood back to the lungs to be reoxygenated.

Arteries

The arteries carry blood from the left ventricle of the heart under very high pressure; the strong muscular walls of the arteries facilitate dilation and constriction, depending on the pressure levels. These large-bore vessels then branch off into arterioles, whose function is to regulate the blood flow to the capillary beds. The arterial blood contains a high percentage of erythrocytes (the oxygen-carrying cells), leukocytes (cells that fight infection), and thrombocytes/platelets (cells involved in blood clotting). The remainder is made up of plasma, which contains the nutrients and minerals that are delivered to the tissues. Hormones produced by the body are carried in the blood to their target organs, and waste products are carried to the liver and kidneys.

Capillaries

Capillaries consist of a single layer of endothelial cells that are permeable and exist in a complex network. Due to a pressure gradient, they allow diffusion of oxygen and nutrients from the blood into the surrounding tissues. These capillary beds form the conduit between the arterial and venous systems. Capillaries facilitate intracellular waste removal through diffusion, returning waste products back to the venules and veins.

Veins

Veins carry blood back to the heart. Venous blood is deoxygenated, and contains toxins from cell metabolism. It needs to be detoxified and reoxygenated quickly to help maintain homeostasis. Blood returns to the heart through vessels of increasing diameter, with no active pump to facilitate this venous return. To compensate for the tendency of the blood to pool in the most distal palmar and plantar areas, the venous vessels instead contain semilunar valves that have anti-gravitational action, supporting the flow proximally. They also have compressible qualities, so they can tolerate the pressure exerted by the surrounding skeletal muscles. In fact, the movements of the skeletal muscles act to compress the vessels, assisting and facilitating venous return. This is a feature replicated by some of the techniques used in massage. The veins are often situated in close proximity to the main arterial vessels, whose pumping action can also facilitate blood flow to the heart through the veins. However, the speed of flow of the blood returning via venous return is restricted by the bore size of the vessel.

Changing internal pressures in the thoracic region as a result of the action of the diaphragm and intercostal muscles facilitates inhalation and exhalation, and also assists the flow of the venous blood back to the heart. This, too, can be affected positively by appropriate massage, assisting deep 'lateral' breathing, and aiding efficient and significant pressure changes. Thus massage can play an important role in enhancing delivery of pain-reducing hormones, such as endorphins, by aiding venous flow (**45**).

Lymphatic system

The function of the lymphatic system is to provide defence and fight against infection and disease. It is a vast network of capillaries, thin vessels, nodes, ducts, and organs that helps to drain tissues and return fluid to the cardiovascular system via major veins near the heart. Unlike the circulatory system, it is not a closed system, as it begins peripherally in a network of blind capillaries, and ends centrally at the thoracic duct. It acts as a supporting system for the circulatory system, or as a secondary cleansing system. The only

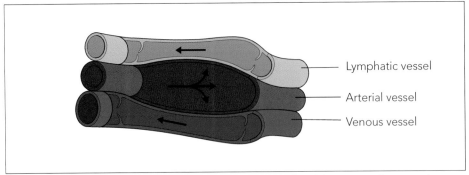

Lymphatic vessel

Arterial vessel

Venous vessel

45 Diagram to show the positive effect the muscular walls of the arteries have on the return flow of both the venous and lymphatic systems. The arrows depict the flow within the different vessels. (Note the semilunar valves within the lymphatic and venous blood vessels.)

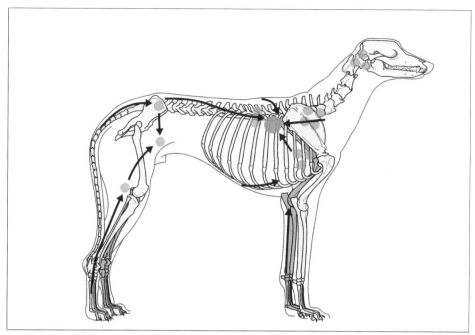

46 The lymphatic system of the dog, showing the main nodes.

direct connection between the two occurs when the lymphatic system drains fluid into the venous system through two ducts near the heart; however, the two systems usually run in parallel.

The fluid that the lymphatic system transports is called lymph. Lymph is similar to blood plasma, although it does not contain red blood cells. Among other things, it contains waste materials, white blood cells, and cancer cells, if these are present. The system has numerous nodes which filter the lymph. The nodes also produce lymphocytes, a type of white blood cell, which fight disease. The circulatory system can only cope with a certain amount of waste products. Excess waste drains into the lymphatic system where the pressure is lower than that of the blood system. If waste particles are too large for the blood system, they are extracted by the lymph vessels, which have larger pores. The lymph collected throughout the body drains into the venous system through the thoracic and jugular ducts (**46**). Lymph originates from the blood, passes through the venous capillary walls and is situated interstitially; it is then absorbed through the cellular walls of the lymphatic capillary network and into the lymphatic system, where it is returned to the venous circulation.

Lymph nodes, where the lymph is filtered, play a crucial part in the body's immune system. Harmful substances which are not neutralized in one node can be carried to the next successive node, where the lymph will again be filtered. Lymphocyte activity in the nodes increases when an infection is present; hence, the lymph nodes become swollen and painful. Phagocytic leucocytes remain in the lymph nodes, destroying harmful substances *in situ*. Also, antibodies produced by different lymphocytes are released into the lymph and circulate in the lymph and the bloodstream.

As in the venous system, the lymphatic system does not have an intrinsic pump and, in similar fashion to the venous system, relies on secondary mechanisms to elicit effective drainage. Again, the skeletal muscles play a large role in effecting this. Like the venous system, the lymphatic system contains small semilunar values to prevent back flow. Also, the adjacent arteries and veins assist with the distal to proximal flow. As with blood flow, pressure changes within the thoracic cavity are important for continuing lymphatic movement. Therefore, when a dog is active and there is good skeletal muscular movement, the system can work efficiently, aiding adequate detoxification.

Massage can influence the lymphatic system effectively, especially in the veteran dog, or one with impaired mobility. This could be used to great effect post-operatively, when movement is restricted; also, the effective removal of post-anaesthetic toxins could aid a fast recovery. In some cases of lymphoedema, appropriate massage can ease the symptoms by assisting drainage, using gentle massage over the most proximal lymphatic node to where the swelling is at its most exaggerated, and then applying light and gentle effleurage (a form of massage), working proximally from the isolated lymph node.

In conclusion, the lymphatic system plays a very important role in the body's defence system. Working alongside the venous system it forms a vital cleaning system for the body, without which homeostasis would not be possible and other systems, such as the musculature, would be compromised.

Comparative human and canine anatomy

Comparative anatomy of the human and dog is an in-depth and precise science; however, for the purpose of this chapter, it has been simplified into areas that are relevant to our area of study. Although studying the differences between the human and the dog is not essential, it is widely accepted by many practitioners as being extremely interesting and helpful. In fact, studying and treating humans can provide a greater insight into applying physical therapy and understanding physiology and anatomy. A human can provide verbal feedback and can be requested to lie still; also, so much more is visible when the skin is not covered in fur. By looking at both the human and dog, one can learn the many similarities between the two species and how they differ. For example, skeletally, all mammals look quite similar. However, a dog can jump proportionally much higher than a horse; to understand how this is possible, and how a dog moves, can give a practitioner a greater knowledge in order to provide effective treatment.

The easiest way to visualize the differences between a canine and a human skeleton is to 'crush' the human ribs to form an angulated sternum and then place the scapulae adjacent and opposite on the sagittal plane (**47**). The obvious difference between the two is that a human has a plantigrade stance (we take the body's weight on the plantar surface of our feet), whereas a dog's stance is digitigrade, meaning they bear weight on their

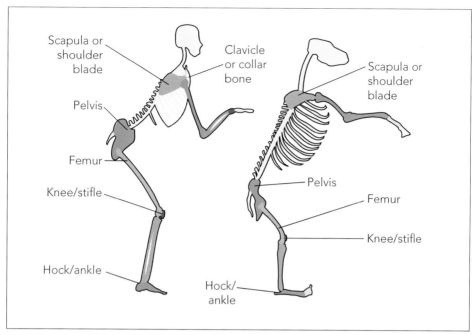

47 Comparison between dog (digitigrade) and human (plantigrade) skeletons.

phalanges or digits. Due to the dog being a quadruped and the human a biped, weight transference and mobility is reflected within the foundation and supporting structures of the body. Most joints allow movement through more than one plane; however, the dog's most obvious limitations are through the joints providing movement through the dorsal and ventral planes (adduction and abduction), and some rotational movements through the transverse plane.

Appendicular skeleton

Thoracic limb

Scapula

The scapula in the dog supports the main muscles used for support, mobility, and weightbearing while in motion and when static. It also receives and dissipates concussion. The potential movement of the scapula can be defined by its orientation and angulation with the thoracic cage. The spines of the scapulae lie at an angle of approximately 35° on the transverse plane, which naturally differs according to breed or type, and therefore intended use. Its attachment to the axial skeletal is solely by soft tissue and its design and role constitutes a major difference between the two species.

The human scapular spine lies on the same relative transverse plane, at 45°; however, due to the free movement required of the arm in the transverse lateral/medial plane, extra stability is required which is facilitated by the clavicle. The dog does not possess a clavicle in the form that a human does and instead, for shoulder stability and strength, it possesses a truncated clavicle in the form of an oval cartilaginous structure that does not articulate with the rest of the skeleton. It spans approximately 1 cm and is located at the tendinous intersection of the brachiocephalicus muscle, in approximately the same anatomical position as the human clavicle.

Humerus

In relation to its human counterpart, the dog has an altered thoracic limb structure to manage its weight and any concussion properties required. The proximal humerus has a more flattened head than that of the human, and distally has a well-defined olecranon fossa and supratrochlear foramen for securing the anconeal process of the ulna; this is crucial for shoulder stability. This is a problematic area for many breeds, as this is a contributory factor in elbow dysplasia; the humerus in the achondroplastic breeds is often bowed to facilitate the shoulder assembly.

There are basically three types of front assemblies in the dog, and these can be used to define the use of a dog. The achondroplastic type are short-legged dogs such as a Dachshund or some Jack Russell terriers; these have shortened limbs, often with valgus or varus lower limb (bowed through carpal growth discrepancy) but have a good angulation between scapula and humerus required for digging. Greyhounds and Lurchers have a less pronounced shoulder angulation than the achondroplastic dog, lending itself to speed. The third type is the dog intended for retrieving or herding work, where the most distal part of the humerus should align with the most caudal aspect of the dorsal scapula region. This angulation is intended for good muscle attachment to provide balance and strength.

Ulna

The ulna in most breeds is the longest bone in the dog. It possesses a large and prominent olecranon process, forming the point of the elbow. This is designed to hold the powerful and supporting triceps brachii muscle group, which are stabilizing and anti-gravitational.

Carpal joints

The carpal joints in the human and canine contain the same number of bones, but in the canine, two are fused and they have a slightly differing construction. In the human, the retinaculum across the palmar side of the wrist draws the outer bones of the wrist together, thus forming a well-defined 'tunnel'; this forms a housing for the tendons and median nerve (when the median nerve is compromised, carpal tunnel syndrome ensues). The dog possesses the same number of carpal bones but the arrangement is altered, with the radial carpal bone parallel to the fused scaphoid and lunate bones.

Axial skeleton

Vertebral column
The vertebral formula is different in the human and the dog:
Canine: C7, T13, L7, S3 (fused), caudal (CA) or coccyx 15–21.
Human: C7, T12, L5, S5 (fused), coccyx 3–4.

Costals
The costals are small bones that articulate with the thoracic vertebrae in both the dog and the human, providing protection for the heart and lungs within the thoracic chamber. In the dog (to a greater extent than in the human), they also help support the shoulder assembly through extrinsic muscular connections; in the dog, this provides stability and fluidity through costal movement when it is in motion.

Pelvis
The fused ilium, ischium, and pubis bones comprise the pelvis, with the ischium providing a wide and broad projection caudally to support the massive hamstring muscle group that is required for propulsion and elevation. The pelvis of the dog is a different shape to that of the human; it is smaller and narrower, and lies within the transverse and dorsal planes.

The commonality between the species is that they both possess a muscular system to suit their function. This means that they both have deep supporting muscles that ensure the stability of the axial skeleton, which enables the appendicular skeleton to be appropriately supported and stabilized too. This can also ensure that the joints become efficient and economical levers, providing sustained movement to the whole.

Pelvic limbs
The femur is the heaviest and largest bone in the dog, whereas the ulna is the longest; in the human, the longest bone is the femur. The stifle is constructed in the same configuration as in the human knee, both relying on good conformation for stability. Muscular stability is provided through the pelvis, plus tendons and ligaments that provide integrity to the joint. The calcaneous of the dog is almost identical to the human ankle (calcaneous) bone, both supporting the Achilles tendon. The canine tarsus contains the same number of bones as the human's, being similar to the human ankle. However, as with the palmar surface of the thoracic limb, the plantar surface of the pelvic limb is the phalanges.

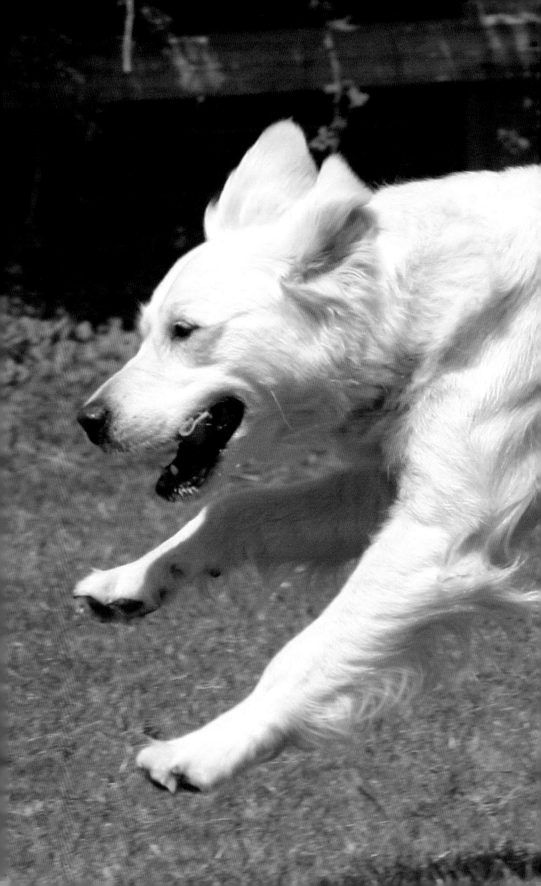

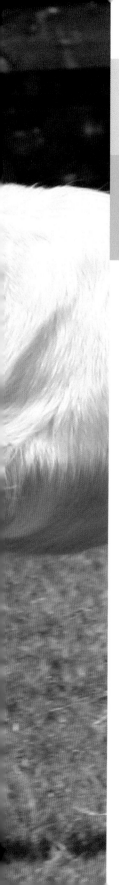

3

How a Dog Moves

Julia Robertson

- Introduction
- Muscle placement and action
- Initiation of movement
- Development of the puppy

Introduction

In order for a dog to move, the body relies on an effective interrelationship between its systems, including: a functional muscular system, innervation from the nervous system, the support and articulation of the skeletal system, together with the metabolic transport of the vascular systems. These form the coordination required for a defined patterning and phasing of muscles. If any part of this chain breaks, the movement loses its integrity.

An understanding of myology, with regards to the placement and action of the individual muscles and muscle groups, is a vital part of the knowledge required when assessing a dog for treatment. It is also important to understand how muscles work together to provide the different actions. This is significant because, in order to treat a dog successfully, an assessment has to be made to identify where a break in that chain may have occurred and what the resultant effects may be.

The kinetic chain

To look at the system from an engineering or mechanical perspective, it is a complex pattern of simple levers and pulleys which needs to accommodate a wide variety of movement and maintain stability through the movement. These levers or joints are then pulled at slightly different angles, according to the insertions and origins of the articulating muscles. Therefore, for them to phase together to form a stable and coordinated action, and cope with the additional stresses caused by gravity (downward pressure), is an intricate and exacting process.

Biomechanics is an extremely complex area of science, and this section does not intend to describe it in detail, but to give an overview on how basic movement is initiated and executed. This chapter will not specify the list of muscles and their involvement with different actions, just the main individuals and/or groups.

Muscle placement and action

Pelvic region

The main drive of the dog comes from the pelvic limbs, relying on the power of the hip flexors and extensors to power the dog forwards. The forward momentum travels through the lumbar and thoracic regions, then uses the thoracic limbs to steer and direct, while receiving the concussion through the recoil system of the shoulder and carpus. Like any finely-tuned engine, the dog requires a huge degree of balance and stability. When looking at the skeletal aspects, the impetus drives through the sacroiliac joint together with the ventral flexion of the lumbar region (**48**). This works in unison with flexion and extension of the femur, which acts as a massive lever through the coxofemoral (hip) joint, driving the forward movement, and at the same time demanding stability and balance through the pelvis. The coxofemoral joint can provide both flexion and extension and a degree of adduction and abduction. Therefore, the integrity of this joint has to be at an optimum state to receive and transmit the forces, together with the extreme pressures being exerted.

The muscular power and drive provided to these levers and joints comes from the hip flexors and extensors. However, without all the moving structures being adequately supported by the postural muscles, they will not withstand the energy and forces created, and optimal range of movement and versatility will not be achieved.

The deep postural muscles of the hip joint (**49**) are:

- m. obturator internus and externus.
- mm. gemelli.
- m. quadratus femoris.
- m. middle gluteal (**50**).
- m. deep gluteal (**50**).
- m. piriformis.

These muscles are critical for stability and balance within the coxofemoral joint. Even with perfect joint congruence, imbalance can result from inappropriate development, exercise, injury, or all three.

The resultant imbalance from this joint may not remain within the joint itself; it can also, through a chain of disparity, lead to weakness within the stifle. There may also be the further complication of thoracic limb compensation. Stability of this joint will naturally occur if a young dog is offered the appropriate amount and type of exercise, if it has no other injuries. Conversely, excessive or inappropriate exercise can also cause problems, both skeletally and muscularly. Consequently, as far as any kinetic chain is concerned, full stability and balance within the 'axle' (the pelvis) is profound and, without this, full and consistent function will never be reached.

48 Important joints in the pelvic region for movement.
1: Sacroiliac joint;
2: Area of coxofemoral joint (Courtesy of Henry Robertson.)

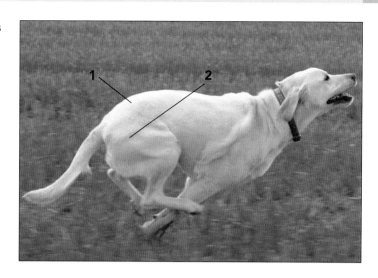

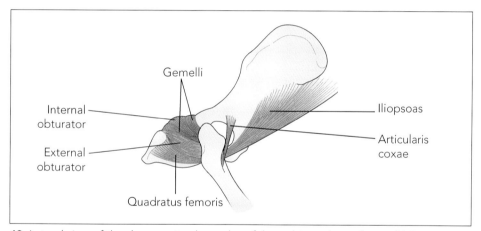

Gemelli

Internal obturator

External obturator

Quadratus femoris

Iliopsoas

Articularis coxae

49 Lateral view of the deep postural muscles of the pelvis and coxofemoral joint.

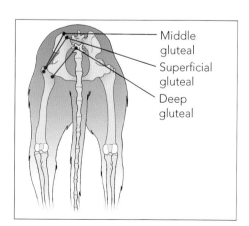

Middle gluteal
Superficial gluteal
Deep gluteal

50 Cranial view of the croup muscle group attachments.

Initiation of movement

Before any movement is initiated, the region has to be stabilized, or the body will not have sufficient resistance to enable movement. A major stabilizer within the pelvic/lumbosacral region is the m. rectus abdominis, which joins the thorax and the pelvis ventrally. This muscle (plus other deep lumbar muscles) provides part of the crucial balance and support through the lumbar region. It also aids dorsal flexion of the pelvis, along with the other hip flexors. On a dog with a short or close coat, a clear abdominal line can be seen when the muscle contracts (**55**).

CASE STUDY 4

Monty, a 5-year-old Border Collie, was rescued from living in one room. He had had no exercise during his young and developing years, and had spent most of his time lying on a windowsill looking out of the window. His stance suggested that there was some form of pelvic and stifle incongruity. The radiographs showed excellent hip and stifle formation (**51, 52**). However, if his gluteal region is studied, this area is underdeveloped, indicating a lack of juvenile stimulation (**53**).

With a combination of massage therapy, hydrotherapy, and neural pathway stimulation, his stability, shape, and balance improved markedly (**54**). Please note: In the case of a dysplastic dog, or one with a femoral head and neck excision, then exercises to create muscular balance within the joint will assist enhanced joint movement through stabilization of the ineffectual joint with balanced intrinsic pelvic muscles (**49, 50**).

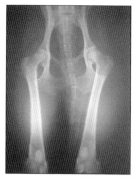
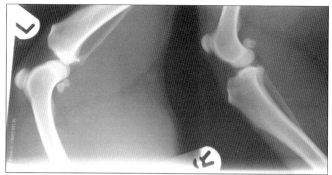

51, 52 Radiographs of Monty, demonstrating good pelvic and stifle construction.

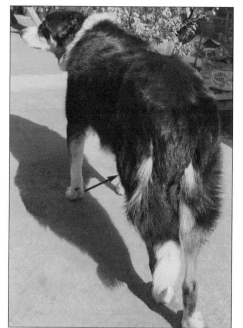
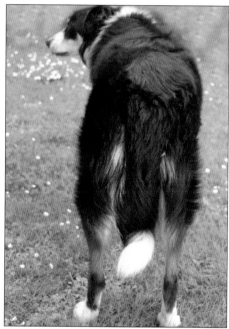

53 Monty showing lack of gluteal development before treatment (arrow).

54 Monty after treatment and physical therapy, showing some improved pelvic stability and gluteal development.

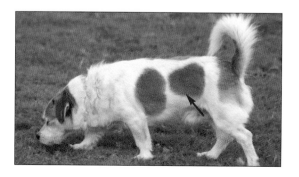

55 Abdominal lift. (arrow)

Planes motion

A plane in this context is an imaginary straight line drawn between two points (**56**).

- Frontal plane – divides the body and limbs longitudinally into two equal right and left halves.
- Sagittal plane – divides the body and limbs parallel to the medial plane.
- Transverse plane – divides the body at right angles through the body's axis.

Forward movement in the sagittal plane (flexion and extension)

Protraction of the pelvic joint

Protraction is when the limb is drawn forwards (**57**). This defines stride length and involves flexion of the hip and stifle. When movement is initiated, the abdominals concentrically contract to assist stabilization and flexion of the lumbar region. The mm. gluteal assist

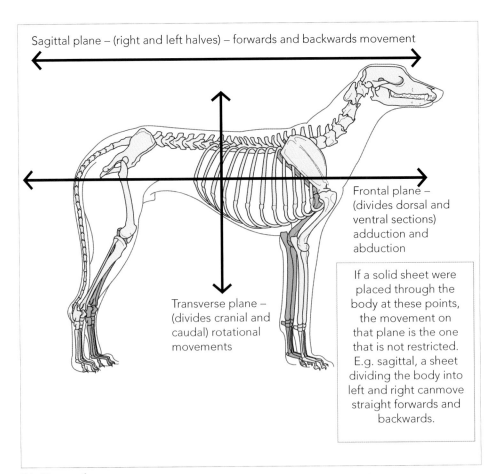

Sagittal plane – (right and left halves) – forwards and backwards movement

Frontal plane – (divides dorsal and ventral sections) adduction and abduction

Transverse plane – (divides cranial and caudal) rotational movements

If a solid sheet were placed through the body at these points, the movement on that plane is the one that is not restricted. E.g. sagittal, a sheet dividing the body into left and right canmove straight forwards and backwards.

56 Planes of movement.

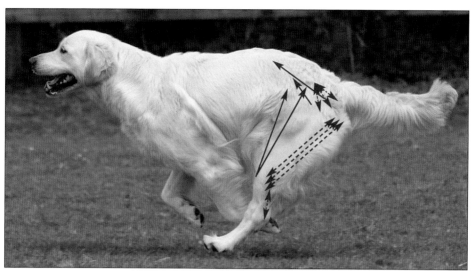

57 Protraction of the pelvic limb, showing concentric contraction (solid arrows) and eccentric contraction (broken arrows). (The adductors, lying medially to the pelvic limb, are not shown.) (Courtesy of Henry Robertson.)

stabilization of the coxofemoral region through eccentric contraction. The m. longissimus lumborum stabilizes the vertebrae. *Table* 3 presents the main muscles that contract concentrically and eccentrically.

The m. psoas major and m. iliacus play a crucial role in pelvic flexion, again forming a linkage between the thoracic and pelvic/femoral regions. Assisting the protraction is the quadricep group, together with the mm. sartorius and m. tensor fascia latae. The adductors lying medially to the femur also support the action by preventing the limb abducting when on the point of balance and transition. The dynamic ability for eccentric contraction of the gluteal muscular group and the hamstring muscular group plays a crucial part in affecting a full range of movement.

Table 3 Muscles involved in protraction of the pelvic joint

Concentric contraction
m. iliopsoas
m. tensor fascia latae (tenses the
 fascia latae)
m. psoas major
m. iliacus
quadricep group
mm. sartorius (caudal and cranial)

Eccentric contraction
gluteal group
hamstring group (m. biceps femoris,
m. semitendinosus, and
m. semimembranosus)
m. gastrocnemius

Retraction of the pelvic joint

The pelvic limb is retracted when the foot hits the ground and the body is projected forwards and there is extension in the hip, stifle, and hock (**58**). This action requires integral stability through the pelvis to both support the weight of the dog and enable the body to thrust forward. The stability is supplied by eccentric contraction of the m. rectus abdominis, the adductor group, m. gracilis, and the deep and medial gluteal muscles. *Table 4* presents the main muscles involved in retraction of the pelvic limb.

This movement is performed effectively if the eccentrically contracting muscles perform optimally. In order to perform a maximum range of movement, stability is the key. Any lack of integrity is not going to allow a dog to gallop, which is where one foot is needed to complete the follow-through; at a gallop, before initiation of protraction, there is one pelvic limb fully weightbearing. The gluteal group is also stabilizing and concentrically contracting, assisting protraction along with the adductor group and gracilis.

Table 4 Muscles involved in retraction of the pelvic limb

Concentric contraction
m. biceps femoris
m. semimembranosus
m. semitendinosus
m. gracilis (to a degree)
m. superficial gluteal
m. gastrocnemius
adductor group (to a degree depending on the plane of movement)

Eccentric contraction
m. iliopsoas
m. tensor fascia latae (supports the fascia latae)
m. psoas major
m. iliacus
quadricep group
mm. sartorius (caudal and cranial)
mm. adductor group (to a degree, depending on plane of movement)

Thoracic region

The thoracic limb is held onto the main part of the body by muscle alone; there are no bony attachments assisting the stability (**59**). The vulnerability is evident, however, as although requirements for the absorption of concussion are well met in normal situations, the muscles are highly susceptible to overuse.

The thoracic limbs are intended to give direction, receive concussion, and support the proportionally heaviest part of the dog through all types of movement, including jumping. Their structure accommodates the many different movements and direction changes required through the soft tissue attachments and the recoil action of the carpal joints. Like the pelvic limb, the thoracic limb protracts, retracts, and can perform abduction and adduction to a limited degree. Most of these movements involve the scapula and its muscular attachments (**60**). The size and shape of the scapula indicate the importance of this flat bone; its large flat surface allows the pennate muscles to attach. It also has exaggerated processes, which are required for the strong fusiform muscles to attach to.

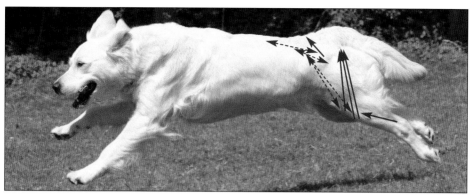

58 Retraction of the pelvic limb showing concentric contraction (solid arrows) and eccentric contraction (broken arrows). (Courtesy of Henry Robertson.)

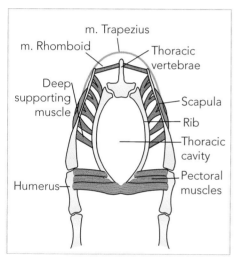

59 Muscles attaching the thoracic limb to the thorax (the shoulder sling).

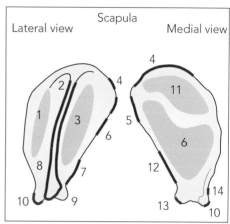

60 Lateral and medial aspects of the scapula showing areas of muscle attachment (in grey block or black solid lines). 1: Supraspinatus; 2: trapezius and deltoid; 3: infraspinatus; 4: rhomboideus; 5: teres major; 6: subscapularis; 7: teres minor and long head of triceps; 8: omotransversarius; 9: deltoideus; 10: biceps brachii; 11: serratus ventralis; 12: long head of triceps; 13: teres minor; 14: coracobrachialis.

As with the pelvic limb, the postural muscles play an active and crucial role in the whole function of the limb (*Table 5*). These muscles are both medial and lateral to the scapula and are extrinsic to the limb. The thoracic limb also has an important relationship with the neck, as much of the thoracic limb movement involves muscular connections within the cervical region. Therefore, the afore-mentioned stresses and strains will also affect the cervical region. Many of the postural muscles are also involved with flexion, extension, adduction, and abduction of the limb.

The main fixing of the scapula is to the thoracic cage; this is not a static attachment, as has been demonstrated cineradiographically by Rachel Page Elliott. Also, the scapula is expected to swing, at a moderate trot, through a movement plane of 30° (measured by the degree of movement from the cranial to dorsal border of the scapula); at a gallop or canter, this angle would increase.

Unlike the pelvic limb that has a firm fixing through the pelvis, the thoracic limb does not have this firm fixing, yet the flexibility and the planes of movement expected are equal. Also, the weight-bearing potential is greater. There is much talk of shoulder angulation, especially within different breed standards; however, this is something that is not of real concern to the kinetic chain, as, whatever the angle movement, it can present similar problems. However, if bad conformation or disproportionate angulations are present, it will impact negatively on the robust quality of the gait.

Protraction of the shoulder

Protraction of the shoulder occurs when the scapula is drawn caudally and the limb is drawn cranially (**61**). Note the extreme bulge over m. supraspinatus. *Table 6* presents the main muscles involved in protraction of the shoulder.

Table 5 Deep postural muscles of the scapula

m. subscapularis
m. serratus ventralis
m. rhomboideus (to a degree)
m. pectoral (deep, in conjunction with the m. serratus ventralis)
m. infraspinatus
m. supraspinatus
m. biceps brachii
triceps group (form tension and stability through the joint when standing)

Table 6 Muscles involved in protraction of the shoulder

Concentric contraction
m. trapezius (thoracic)
m. rhomboideus major and minor (elevating and drawing scapula towards the trunk)
m. subscapularis
m. serratus ventralis – thoracic pectoral group (during weight trans-ference)
m. cleidobrachialis
m. supraspinatus
m. omotransversarius

Eccentric contraction
triceps group
m. latissimus dorsi (initially)
m. trapezius (cervical)
m. serratus ventralis – cervical
mm. teres (minor and major)
m. infraspinatus

61 Protraction of the shoulder (note the hypertonia within m. supraspinatus) showing concentric contraction (solid arrows) and eccentric contraction (broken arrows). (Courtesy of Henry Robertson)

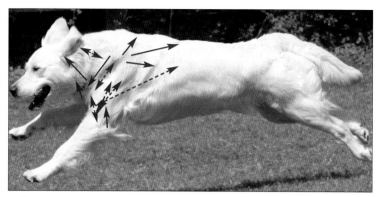

To initiate protraction of the thoracic limb, the scapula has to be elevated so as to lift the leg off the ground. This is facilitated by the m. trapezius and m. rhomboideus, supported by the m. serratus ventralis, m. subscapularis, and m. deep pectoralis. The dorsal portion of the scapula then is drawn caudally by the m. trapezius (thoracic section); the m. omotransversarius and m. cleidobrachialis consequently draw the ventral section of the scapula cranially, producing the angulation of the scapula required for protraction.

To flex the shoulder so that the leg can extend involves mm. teres major and minor, m. infraspinatus, the scapular and acromial sections of the m. deltoideus; the m. latissimus dorsi draws the trunk forwards and assists flexion of the shoulder. Flexion of the elbow is instigated by the m. biceps brachii and m. brachialis. The shoulder and elbow then extend into full protraction; this involves m. supraspinatus, m. infraspinatus (to a small degree), m. cleidobrachialis, m. omotransversarius, and the extensor group of the limb. The paw will hit the ground using the metacarpal pad, then roll forwards into a point of 'break-over' where the line of balance is driven forwards onto the digital pads before they leave the ground. This should be a smooth, rounded, and level movement, but it can easily be compromised by:

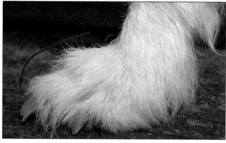

62 Long claws.

- Excessively long nails (often overlooked) (**62**).
- Pain in the phalanges.
- Amputation of a digit.
- Carpal trauma or chronic disease.

Long nails assert an upward force on the phalanges and inhibit a smooth break-over motion of the dog's foot.

Transition from protraction to retraction

During the transition between protraction and retraction, the extended limb forms a solid 'column' to support the weight of the dog. The triceps brachii group is initially in eccentric contraction, then, as the limb drives forward, it transfers into concentric contraction to extend the elbow, assisting the forward drive action, along with the m. pectoralis (deep and superficial parts), m. serratus ventralis, m. infraspinatus, m. supraspinatus, m. deltoideus, and the teres group (63).

This transition, and the propulsion of the trunk cranially, requires a complex system of support, coupled with an almost 'locked' pivoting mechanism. This is provided through the shoulder and elbow joints; these will maintain balance and provide enough strength to sustain forward trajectory. Flexibility of the hyperextension and then the recoil actions of the carpus is critical to the smooth conversion from protraction to retraction (see 61). For full retraction, the m. latissimus dorsi and m. triceps brachii are at full contraction, supported by the extrinsic muscles of the scapula (the rhomboideus and the cervical section of the trapezius muscles). These are assisted by the m. serratus ventralis and the pectoral group of muscles.

Retraction of the shoulder

Retraction of the shoulder is when the scapula is drawn cranially and the limb caudally (64). *Table 7* presents the main muscles involved in retraction of the shoulder.

The neck

Much of the support of the head and neck comes from the ligamentum nuchae or nuchal ligament, which consists of paired

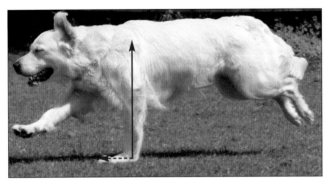

63 Transition between protraction and retraction. 'Locking' of shoulder and elbow (solid arrow). Hyperextension of the carpus (broken arrow). (Courtesy of Henry Robertson)

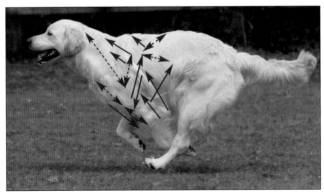

64 Retraction of the shoulder, showing concentric contraction (solid arrows) and eccentric contraction (broken arrows). (Courtesy of Henry Robertson)

Table 7 Muscles involved in retraction of the shoulder

Concentric contraction
triceps brachii group
m. latissimus dorsi
m. trapezius (cervical)
m. serratus ventralis – (cervical)
m. infraspinatus (depending on point of shoulder extension, providing stabilization)
pectorals
mm. teres (minor and major)
mm. rhomboideus major and minor (elevating and drawing scapula towards the trunk)

Eccentric contraction
m. trapezius (thoracic)
m. subscapularis
m. serratus ventralis – thoracic pectoral group (during weight transference)
m. cleidobrachialis
m. supraspinatus (depending on point of shoulder extension, providing stabilization)
m. infraspinatus (to a small degree)
m. omotransversarius

elastic funiculi nuchae that bridge the cervical vertebrae; it extends from the spine of the axis to the first thoracic spinous process (**65**). Here, it joins with the less elastic supraspinous ligament; this attaches to all the spinous processes of the more caudal vertebrae, up to the third sacral vertebra. The nuchal ligament assists in opposing flexion by its reflexive strength and retraction, saving the dog's muscle energy by sustaining the level of the head and greatly easing the muscular effort of lifting the head when the neck is lengthened, especially when the nose is on the ground (during scenting).

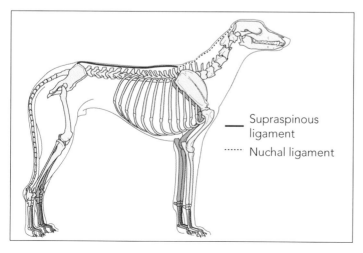

Supraspinous ligament
········ Nuchal ligament

65 The nuchal and supraspinous ligaments.

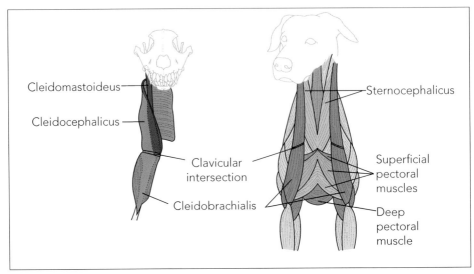

66 Deep muscles of the neck, cranial view.

This remarkable modified apparatus contains more elastic components than other ligaments, as it is a muscle-saving device that is especially important when reacting in a 'fight or flight' situation. Its reflexive qualities save a huge amount of energy that will be needed for running. The muscles that are used in neck movements are (**66**):

- Neck extension – when the neck is stretched upwards with the nose in the air, the following muscles contract:
  m. rhomboideus.
  m. trapezius – cervical section.
  m. splenius.
- Neck flexion – when the neck is bent downwards, allowing the nose to go to the ground, the following muscles contract:
  m. sternohyoideus (crucial role, due to its influence on the tongue).
  m. cleidocephalicus.
  m. sternocephalicus.
  m. omotransversarius.

- Lateral flexion of the neck – when the neck moves the head to the left or the right, the following muscles contract:
  m. cleidocephalicus.
  m. omotransversarius.
  m. splenius.

Vertebral column

Figures **67** and **68** shows some of the muscles involved in vertebral extension. Unilateral concentric contraction of these muscles is a major contributory factor to lateral flexion of the vertebrae. Flexion is assisted by the concentric contraction of several abdominal muscles:

- internal and external obliques.
- major and minor psoas.
- m. iliacus.
- intercostal muscles (to a small degree).
- pectoral group (to a small degree).

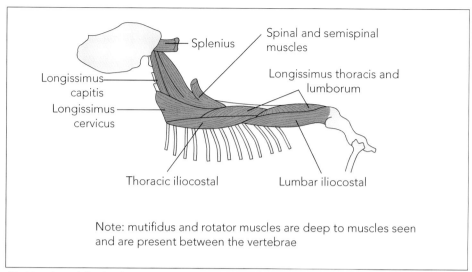

Splenius

Spinal and semispinal muscles

Longissimus thoracis and lumborum

Longissimus capitis

Longissimus cervicus

Thoracic iliocostal

Lumbar iliocostal

Note: mutifidus and rotator muscles are deep to muscles seen and are present between the vertebrae

67 Muscles of the back and neck.

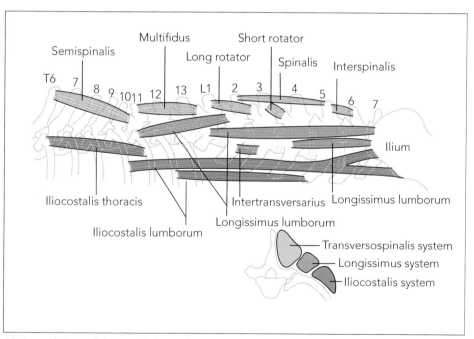

Multifidus   Short rotator

Semispinalis

Long rotator   Spinalis   Interspinalis

T6   7   8   9   1011   12   13   L1   2   3   4   5   6   7

Ilium

Iliocostalis thoracis   Intertransversarius   Longissimus lumborum

Iliocostalis lumborum   Longissimus lumborum

Transversospinalis system

Longissimus system

Iliocostalis system

68 Lateral view of the epaxial muscles.

Movement in the frontal plane (adduction and abduction)

The frontal plane includes both abduction and adduction; a very obvious and typical example of abduction is that of a male dog cocking his pelvic limb; this is abduction of the pelvic limb. Adduction is when the dog draws its pelvic limb closer to the centre line of its body.

Abduction of the pelvic limb

Table 8 presents the main muscles involved in abduction of the pelvic limb. When the pelvic limb moves away from the centre line of the body, the sartorius (caudal and cranial) and tensor fascia lata (TFL) initiate the movement by adding tension to the stifle. Tensing of the m. sartorius and TFL draws the stifle laterally, allowing the superficial and middle gluteal muscles to continue the movement.

Adduction of the pelvic limb

Table 9 presents the main muscles involved when the pelvic limb moves towards the central line of the body. The muscles of adduction are more defined than those for abduction; this is because the lateral forces when running in the sagittal plane are great and the need for stability and the restraint of extreme abduction are constant.

Abduction of the thoracic limb

This is when the thoracic limb moves away from the central line of the body. When a dog moves through a set of weave poles in agility or turns quickly, abduction of the limb is employed as part of the steerage mechanism through this limb. Great stability and flexibility is needed in the front assembly to carry out this manoeuvre. *Table 10* presents the main muscles involved in abduction of the thoracic limb.

The dew claw or medial phalanx gives further stability when the limb is abducting at speed (**69**). When a dog is turning at speed, the lateral force on the thoracic limb is great, and preventing the limb from

---

Table 8 Muscles involved in abduction of the pelvic limb

Concentric contraction
- superficial gluteal
- middle gluteal
- m. piriformis

Eccentric contraction
- adductor group
- m. gracilis
- m. pectineus

Table 9 Muscles involved in adduction of the pelvic limb

Concentric contraction
- adductor group
- m. gracilis
- m. pectineus

Eccentric contraction
- superficial gluteal
- middle gluteal
- m. piriformis

Table 10 Muscles involved in abduction of the thoracic limb

Concentric contraction
- m. trapezius (both cervical and thoracic sections)
- m. supraspinatus (initiates)
- m. infraspinatus
- m. deltoideus (acromion head)
- m. rhomboideus

Eccentric contraction
- m. subscapularis (**59**)
- m. superficial pectoral
- m. coracobrachialis

violently abducting takes a massive amount of static contraction and eccentric contraction by the pectoral group of muscles. Meanwhile, the dew claw acts as an anchor to stabilize the limb.

Adduction of the thoracic limb

Adduction occurs when the thoracic limb moves towards the central line. Adduction and abduction are shown in Figure **70**. *Table 11* presents the main muscles involved in adduction of the thoracic limb. A key point to remember is that the dog's body will adjust to the current situation with its musculoskeletal system. The eyes should always be looking forward; therefore, whatever happens in the rest of the body, the eyes will, as far as possible, remain on a horizontal plane. For efficient movement, the 'working' legs will be drawn to the centre line of the body, whatever the breed, whatever the length of leg. Figure **71** shows a dog with unbalanced movement, in which the stronger leg is moved onto the centre line.

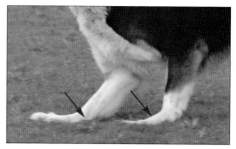

69 The dew claws acting as a crucial anchor during a tight turn.

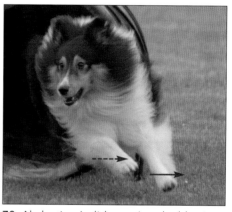

70 Abduction (solid arrow) and adduction (broken arrow) of the thoracic limbs. (Courtesy of Tony LeSigne.)

Table 11 Muscles involved in adduction of the thoracic limb

Concentric contraction
- m. subscapularis
- m. superficial pectoral
- m. coracobrachialis

Eccentric contraction
- m. trapezius (both cervical and thoracic sections)
- m. supraspinatus (initiates)
- m. infraspinatus
- m. deltoideus (acromion head)
- m. rhomboideus

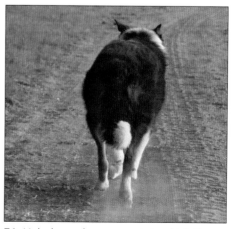

71 Unbalanced movement, in which the dog moves its stronger leg onto the centre line.

Development of the puppy

Early days

When a puppy arrives in its new home and begins its new solitary existence away from other pack members, problems can start developing. In a primal pack, a puppy would not stray far from the den. It would spend its time playing with other members of the pack, exploring the terrain, and slowly developing physically, and also developing a sense of spatial awareness, through climbing on and playing with others (**72**). Food would be brought to it until it was adolescent. Thus, a puppy should not be given a programme of exercise that exceeds its requirement for normal physical development.

Unfortunately, some puppies are exercised inappropriately and allowed to perform extreme movements, such as walking up and down stairs, jumping on and off furniture, and in and out of cars. The concussional effect of these activities on immature joints, joint capsules, and bones is profound. Other, less often considered, forms of inappropriate exercise occur on lead walk: being made to conform to the gait and speed of the handler and, therefore, being unable to develop its own natural gait and speed. This also applies to some working dogs or those that are preparing for other disciplines, such as agility. The type of training the puppy has will have a dramatic effect on its future health and the length of time it can spend in a sport or discipline. Many owners, especially those who have not owned dogs before, or are not educated in puppy development, may be unaware of how fragile puppies are at this age and how any disruptions in a puppy's physical development can result in a future life of diseases, such as osteoarthritis.

Puppies should not be exposed to all the rigours of our environment, as they are developmentally and physiologically unprepared. If the effects of their early activities were immediate, perhaps owners

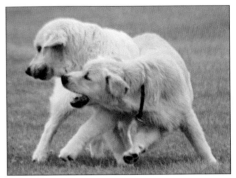

72 Puppies playing naturally, developing their spatial awareness and postural stability. (Courtesy of Liz Pope.)

would act differently, but, unfortunately, they do not appear until a dog is about 7 or 8 years old. If a breed has a propensity to any skeletal conditions, e.g. elbow or hip dysplasia (see Chapter 6), it is extremely advisable to keep high impact exercise to an absolute minimum (see Chapter 7).

Spatial awareness

Spatial awareness is innate but develops through a complexity of actions and working through different planes of movement to develop muscular stability through the stimulation of appropriate muscle patterning. This will include the neural stimulation and proprioceptive awareness of skeletal muscles, especially those involved in postural stability. The requirement for spatial awareness is not just for stability, it is also important for general responsiveness to the surroundings. Many dogs, mainly the giant or large breeds, grow so quickly that they seem unaware of 'where they start and finish'. This can be endearing to humans, but seeing your puppy's legs splaying on the floor indicates that a mobility problem is being stored for the future. Spatial awareness and heightened proprioception are important survival tools and enables a dog to feel secure within its body, which is a significant stress suppressant with psychological and physiological benefits.

To stimulate or 'fire' the appropriate muscles requires specific exercises that encourage activities through various planes of movement; it is critical to start these when the puppy is still developing (**73**). These exercises must be carefully managed, using knowledge of what the puppy is capable of without being overstretched or overtired.

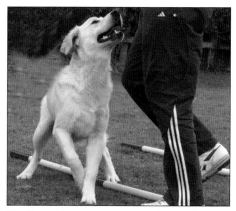

73 Puppy being encouraged to work in the frontal plane – adduction and abduction.

Puppy massage

Puppy massage is an area that has been underdeveloped and one that can serve to benefit puppies and handlers alike (**74**). Massage can facilitate greater bonding and connection between puppy and handler. The owner is able to develop an awareness of their puppy's body map, and will learn what is normal and what is abnormal, e.g. the effects of heat and cold, and so on. The puppy becomes used to being touched, which creates a bond of trust; this is particularly important when veterinary attention is required.

Massage has many direct health benefits. It gently encourages venous return, which in turn encourages arterial delivery to help with growth and cellular development, mineralization of joints, and hormone delivery. It also promotes lymphatic stimulation, which supports the immune system, which is especially important when puppies are in contact with viruses, bacteria, and so on. Massage helps puppies to relax, which aids digestion. Indeed, a study of the biochemical and clinical responses to massage in pre-term human infants showed that post-massage cortisol levels were decreased consistently. Massage

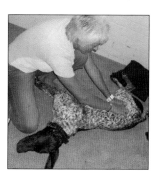

74 Puppy massage class. (Courtesy of Lezleigh Packer.)

encourages the use of neural pathways through physical stimulation and promotes good coordination and spatial awareness through neural and muscular synergy.

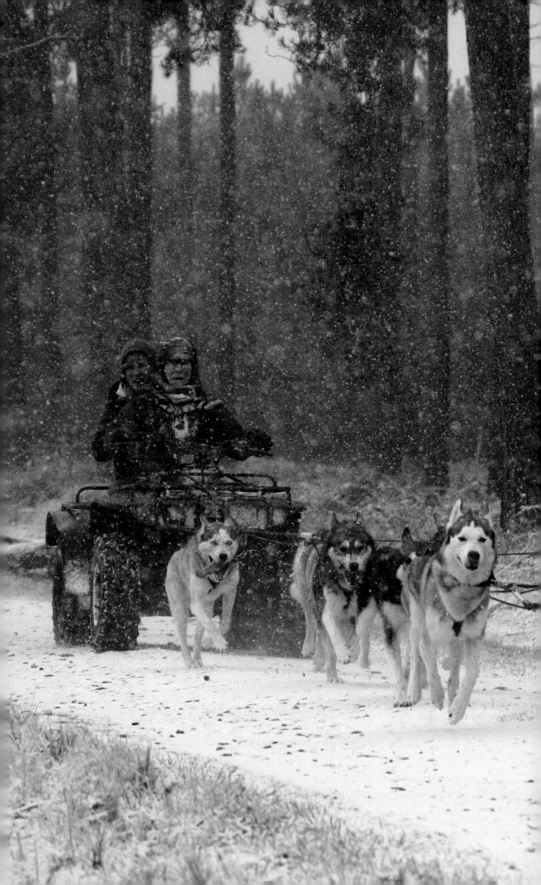

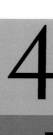

4

Exercise and Activity Preparation

Julia Robertson and Meg Robertson

- Exercise and conditioning
- Performance areas and their stresses
- Warming up and warming down
- Warm-up and warm-down for the handler

Exercise and conditioning

With the canine athlete, training is the part that the majority of dogs and handlers enjoy the most and they devote many hours to it. Teaching a dog to run or jump for performance, even though it is a natural activity, is more complex than is often understood. When preparing for exercise, an area that is not often fully considered is muscle conditioning. There are many activities in which dogs are expected to carry out complex routines with or without apparent high impact, at speed, or with stamina. In many instances, this is done without the benefit of appropriate preparation.

Muscle conditioning

Muscle conditioning and training is key groundwork for any competition or activity. Simple conditioning exercises can promote physiological and organizational changes in the body that will maximize performance and maintain soundness. Appropriate dynamic training will develop neuromuscular coordination and mental discipline. This is a complex subject that involves the appropriate preparation of individual muscle fibres for the onset of sustained activity. Correct conditioning assists the body through enhanced circulation to the muscles which helps to:

• Avoid muscles prematurely fatiguing.
• Cleanse and replenish the fibres post-activity.
• Remove any residual anaerobic by-products.
• Re-establish mineral balance.
• Repair microtrauma in muscle fibre resulting from exercise.

Conditioning includes cardiovascular conditioning (or the enhanced vascularization of muscle fibres), where appropriate training regimes helping to improve blood supply to the muscles required for an intended activity, strength training for increasing power or endurance to targeted muscle groups, and suppling exercises, for developing a range of movement within all joints, creating muscular balance, and reducing the risk of injury.

Good conditioning is developed by well-designed programmes involving appropriate:

• Warm-ups: dynamic exercises that will engage the main global muscles, gradually increasing in activity levels that also incorporate the warming of deeper areas and stabilizing muscles.

This is when an appropriate massage with passive movement can be incorporated (see Chapter 6).

• Sets: groups of combined exercises with rest in between.
• Repetition: performing an exercise several times.
• Progression: choosing the number of sets and repetitions that is appropriate for the age, condition, and fitness of the dog.
• Warm-downs: a dynamic warm-down facilitates the gentle redistribution of blood away from the muscle to the core, assists lactate removal, and assists muscle microfibre repair. This should also include gentle suppling exercises, such as passive movement to ease muscle tension and assist any realigned or displaced fibres; again, an appropriate massage can assist with this process (see Chapter 6).

Length of pace

The 'range' employed by the joint to facilitate movement can also make a significant difference to muscle performance, and this also has a great effect on the strength that can be exerted by a muscle.

Long, or outer range is when a joint moves through its full range, with the agonist and antagonist working at full stretch, using elastic recoil and forward motion to form rhythm and momentum at speed. This is a highly economical function, and it is easier for the fit dog to maintain for speed, but not so much for endurance, e.g. agility dogs, racing Greyhounds, and luring Whippets.

Middle range is when the joints are working at their most efficient for both strength and motion, e.g. Huskies sledding, and Staffordshire Bull Terriers weight-pulling.

Inner range is where the angle of movement is small and forward motion is limited and controlled; this is highly fatiguing due to the stability through core strength and the control through eccentric contraction required, e.g. in obedience work.

Understanding the types of movement that a dog needs to employ is a vital part of training and conditioning; the fact that a slow pace has a high energy requirement is often widely overlooked. Considering the planes of movement (see Chapter 7) that dogs have to use is another factor that is often overlooked. For example, in the case of the agility dog, consider the types of movement, and the rapid changes that are expected from the sagittal to the transverse planes. Repetitive strain injuries may result from many activities during training, competition, and exercising. Flexing of the whole vertebral column in a sustained controlled manner may result from many activities, such as obedience tests, continual jumping and turning, or exercise and training programmes using ball or frisbee throwing and tugging.

Muscular leverage

Performance levels are greatly affected by muscular strength, power, and endurance, which are themselves dependent on the amount of leverage produced by the muscles through the joints. 'Strength' is the greatest amount of force that a muscle can produce in a single maximal effort, e.g. when performing a jump, agility, working trials, and so on. 'Power' is the rate of force generated in pulling exercises, e.g. weight pulling, and Husky sledding. 'Endurance' is the ability to perform repeated contractions before the local muscles fatigue, e.g. during Husky sledding and Canicross.

Muscular balance – postural and core stability

To ensure optimum performance from a dog, its muscles must be 'balanced'. Muscular balance relates to all the muscle groups having the ability to contract and relax, allowing controlled coordination of the muscles, with full range of movement. One important factor to consider when assessing balance is the dog's core stability. The core muscles are those that hold the 'core' – the thoracic and lumbar vertebrae, in a secure balanced position, yet allowing flexibility.

In the author's opinion, the core muscles in the dog include:

- Epaxial system:
  - longissimus group (paravertabral).
- Hypaxial system:
  - transverse abdominals.
  - m. rectus abdominus.
  - internal obliques.
  - m. multifidus (see p.79).
  - external obliques.

Core strength is the balance and inter-realtionship between these two groups. Postural muscles are there to support joint action, but they can only do this if the core of the body remains stable. In other words, unless the main frame of the dog is supported well by the core muscles, any subsequent movements will not be balanced or adequately supported. Therefore, if hard exercise or training continues with a lack of core strength, the balance will be severely compromised through lack of foundational strength. Consequently, this lack of core strength and stability will be apparent by the subtle changing of movement patterns. This is when overuse of joints and muscles starts to take its toll, caused by the ensuing incorrect phasing, leading to compensatory actions and subsequent muscle problems. (75). With a well- developed and balanced core, a dog will have the ability to train hard for a discipline and will be less likely to endure muscular injury. Without this core strength, the integrity of the whole musculature would be constantly challenged (see Chapter 3) (76).

One of the main causes of core and postural dysfunction is due to the

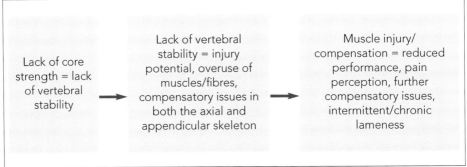

Lack of core strength = lack of vertebral stability	Lack of vertebral stability = injury potential, overuse of muscles/fibres, compensatory issues in both the axial and appendicular skeleton	Muscle injury/ compensation = reduced performance, pain perception, further compensatory issues, intermittent/chronic lameness

Fig 75 Algorithm for core stability and performance.

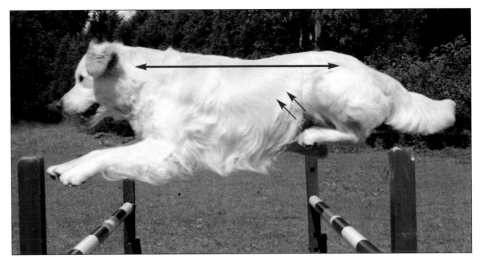

76 As the dog jumps an obstacle wider than his own length, strength is needed within the entire vertebral column, in addition to strength and dynamic force required of the abdominals and obliques (arrows). If these are strong enough, the dog can hold its body in a straight line, almost in a lying down position. (Courtesy of Henry Robertson.)

environment. It can happen when the dog is a puppy or an adolescent; this is the time that the initial core and postural strength should be established. Unfortunately, this is when inappropriate actions and exercise prevent proper development (see Chapter 3). There are many situations that will encourage inappropriate development; the most common is excessive exercise. A puppy does not need long walks; however, it does need stimulation, like scenting exercises in a confined area. These will mentally tire it, but won't put excessive pressure on the joints. Another example preventing most puppies from developing proper postural stability and spatial awareness is the lack of 'natural exercise' that they would get in a pack situation. This type of play would involve scrambling over and wrestling with each other, developing stability through recruiting natural movements in the sagittal, transverse, and frontal planes. Finally, physical problems at home may cause inappropriate development, like the dog being given a bed or cage that is too small, being allowed to go up and down stairs, or having inappropriate high-impact training. This behaviour is then perpetuated when the puppy becomes an adult. It is allowed to jump into and out of cars and on and off furniture or other high objects. This type of repetitive activity can correspond to that of a computer worker or driver who develops bad posture through work and, as a result, suffers from neck and shoulder problems.

Hodges and Richardson (1996, see Further Reading), showed that the cocontraction of the transverse abdominal, multifidus, and internal oblique muscles occurs prior to any movement of the limbs. This suggests that these muscles anticipate dynamic forces that may act on the lumbar vertebrae and stabilize the area prior to any movement. For many dogs with lumbar problems, this theory is demonstrated by the fact that the internal obliques and the transverse abdominals are in a hypertrophic state, which is where they are in a constantly supporting condition rather than one that is switching on only when stability in the area is required. This prevents the normal patterning and phasing of muscle, causing a massive disturbance to the balance and subsequent vertebral support through the core. Being inadequately supported leads to pain, lameness, and general imbalance.

The first signs of these problems can be an apparent reluctance to perform. Many times, trainers have said: 'My dog has lost interest in …'. It is unlikely for a dog to lose interest in an activity that previously they found physically and psychologically fulfilling; it is more likely that they hurt.

In some human studies, it has been shown that the nervous system seems to be able to detect a reduced capability to generate a force from a detailed muscle or group of muscles, and when this occurs, more motor neurons are recruited. This apparent compensation can be replaced by recruiting motor units from areas that remain uninjured within the muscle or from other muscles capable of performing the same tasks.

Thus, in humans, the nervous system is extremely efficient at changing the phasing and patterning of muscles to ensure continued movement; this is a basic survival mechanism. The body's systems, including the muscles, are developed so as to feed back information on, and adjust to, the environment, whether internal or external. The body's mechanisms are developed so that the eyes remain level with the horizon; this allows evaluation and preparation for what is being presented so that the muscles can make appropriate movements in response.

Challenges to core stability

Not all humans are built to be athletes, and neither are dogs! There are obvious conformational or structural factors which can affect overall core stability; these can be managed by adjusting a dog's exercise routine or the type of exercise.

Another challenge to core balance is when a dog's foot hits the ground at an unaccustomed angle. This may occur, for example, in the case of an agility dog that may be used to working on a turf surface in the summer, but is suddenly moved into a sand arena when winter starts. In this situation, the piezo-electric charges received through the joints will assert different stresses through joint surfaces. Putting different stresses on muscles can set up dramatic changes in the dog's biomechanical and kinetic systems; this can cause massive problems in the unstable dog. This includes dogs with minor muscular issues involving shoulder or pelvic instability, including mild hip dysplasia; their core would be comprised accordingly. This problem has also been experienced by many handlers who take their dogs to the beach, to give them a change of scene. This is something that can cause lameness in an unbalanced dog, as the sand on the beach can range from hard, dense sand to soft, water-soaked sand. These look the same, but the resistance of the two is radically different. This would be unknown before the dog ran over the surface, but very apparent afterwards.

Core stability and postural strength

The importance of core stability (axial skeleton strength and balance) and postural strength is key to a performance dog and its ability to continue pain-free within a discipline for an extended period. However, sheer exuberance, loyalty, and adrenaline can compensate and mask pain or mild discomfort. Without the appropriate groundwork promoting the development of good core stability, any exercise discipline can result in areas of weakness and subsequent injury, or chronic problems, such as inflammation resulting from constant low-level injury (77).

- Stress or trauma causes muscle tightness resulting in antagonistic weakness
- Inflammation caused through increased areas of tension (piezo-electric changes)
- Areas of tension cause a lack of good circulatory flow resulting in inflammation due to pain receptor stimulation
- Viscosity of surrounding fascia alters due to inflammation, causing restriction of movement, leading to adhesions
- Tension in muscles causes fibre damage, leading to fibrosis and inflammation, then further damage to adjacent tissue occurs
- Microspasm of muscle spindles communicating with Golgi tendon organs act to restrict movement, with subsequent muscle weakness causing compensatory effects

77 Injury cycle.

If a horse were being trained as a showjumper or eventer, one of the first things to be done would be the 'ground work'. A professional rider or trainer would never allow a horse to jump without ensuring their movement over the ground was of a good standard. This would involve basic dressage moves, simple grid work, and good postural working, so as to encourage the horse to drive from his hindquarters, not from the forehand. This is fundamental for anyone involved in equestrian activities, but it does not seem to hold true for all canine activities. Many training programmes only involve working a dog on one plane of movement, in other words, in straight lines; but very few integrate gentle abduction and adduction exercises. These lateral and medial movements are important for creating neural pathways to many of the core and postural muscles. The middle gluteal muscle is one of the key supporting or postural muscles for the coxofemoral joint. When this is unstable, it creates a pronounced lack of stability through the stifle and the lower back, setting up a poor biomechanical movement that is not sustainable.

Other areas of training should involve the development of spatial awareness, i.e. the dog's awareness of where it 'starts and finishes', and, importantly, the ability to lift each of its legs independently and effortlessly when moving (78).

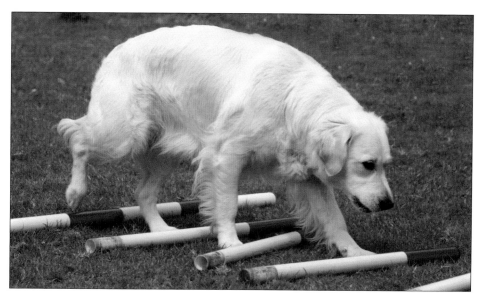

78 A simple exercise where a few poles are laid out in an irregular pattern encourages a dog to concentrate on where to place each foot and when to lift each leg and step over the next pole. (Please note – this is not intended to develop a gait pattern.) (Courtesy of Henry Robertson.)

Appropriate training from all perspectives is critical, whether the dog is a puppy or a rehomed adult. Like all athletes, its muscular health should be continually and professionally assessed to establish the state of balance and tone, and to ensure the correct training programmes are used for the chosen discipline/s. Like all athletes, to prolong a successful career, the canine athlete requires a good team supporting it from all areas of development, fitness, and remedial care (79).

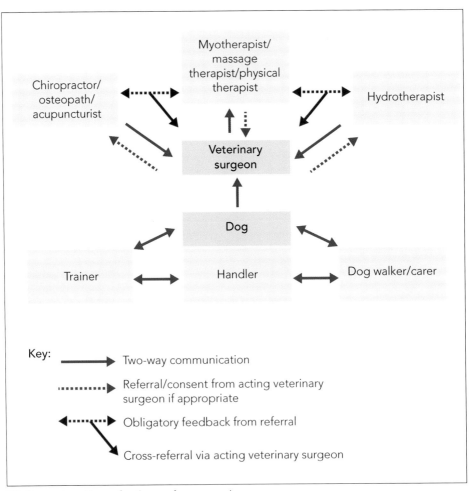

79 Operational team for the performance dog.

Within the canine team, the main player is the dog; everything revolves around its needs and wants. The other key player is the veterinary surgeon. No treatments should ever be applied without their consent or referral; this is a legal requirement and both practitioner and handler will be breaking the law if this is not adhered to.

The team should work cohesively, with good communication. If people run their businesses well, cross-referral and appropriate treatments and therapies will be made widely available to the dog. All practitioners should have a good under-standing of what other therapies can offer, and at what stage of a dog's programme they would be appropriate. Most importantly, any therapist should know immediately when to refer a dog back to its veterinary surgeon.

Performance areas and their stresses

As with human athletes, different disciplines in canine performance have distinct areas of repetitive stress or potential injury. In some cases, a practitioner with good palpation skills can identify the discipline through the tension lines and the length of time that the problem has been going on. In the perfect world, tension should not be evident within a working dog's body. However, to be aware of where the tension is likely to be within an athlete will help treatment and, more importantly, assist a possible change or varying of training, exercise methods, and environmental impacts within key regions. This is not exclusive to performance dogs; many companion dogs have classic repetitive-type strains that can impact heavily on their musculature, causing secondary problems such as arthritis or laxity within joints. These can have repercussions in mid- or later life.

Dogs that perform and have a task, whether it is something true to the breed type, like a gundog retrieving, or a dog that requires the physical and mental stimulation of agility or obedience training, are generally the most satisfied and contented dogs. Because of this dedication to their work, it is often up to the handler, veterinary surgeon, or practitioner to determine when they are fit to perform and when they are not. There is no doubt that when a dog's body is exercised and is put through stresses and endurance it develops good recovery mechanisms, both physiologically and psychologically, which can benefit a dog throughout its life.

Jumping

The requirement for any dog that is involved in any form of jumping is the same:

- Good weightbearing requirement and stability from the thoracic limbs to support the whole body weight at the point of take-off.
- Flexibility through the lumbar region for pelvic and lumbar flexion and extension.
- Stability through the pelvic region to support the upward thrust.
- Uncompromised extensors and flexors of the pelvic region to provide the full range of movement.
- A strong and robust core to sustain the flight and possible twist.
- Good concussional qualities from the thoracic limbs' intrinsic and extrinsic muscles to cope with landing and turning.

The stresses of jumping are dealt with well by a dog, but to achieve high jumping with ease takes flexibility and support from both the thoracic and pelvic areas. The whole process of the jump requires efficient weight transference and uncompromised flexibility through the action of the hip flexors. For the take-off (80), the thoracic region stabilizes the entire thoracic limb through static and eccentric contraction of the m. triceps group. This, combined with other intrinsic and extrinsic muscles, will form a solid column of strength (similar to the 'stay system' of the horse) through the limb, facilitating a 'springboard' take-off. If there is any form of instability in the thoracic limb or shoulder, the dog will falter and hesitate before take-off.

Figure **80** shows the dog one stride before the point of take-off; the weight is transferred to the thoracic region, supporting the flexion of the lumbar and pelvic region. Excellent balance is the key at this point. For the take-off, power in the lumbar region is the key (**81**). The lumbar region is extended through the thrust and force driven through the pelvis by the complete extension of the pelvic limbs. This explosive force causes a recoil of the phalanges on the dog's pelvic limb. In the flight over the jump: stability is important (**82**). This results from good core strength, and balance is required to sustain flight and have the ability to twist and change to another 'plane' mid-flight.

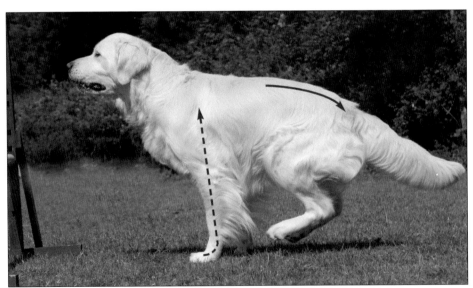

80 Prior to take-off. Solid arrow: flexibility; broken arrow: stability/concussion. (Courtesy of Henry Robertson.)

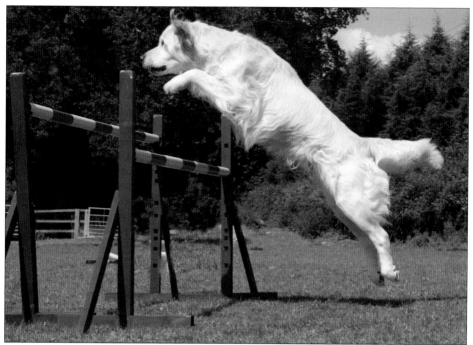

81 Take-off. (Courtesy of Henry Robertson.)

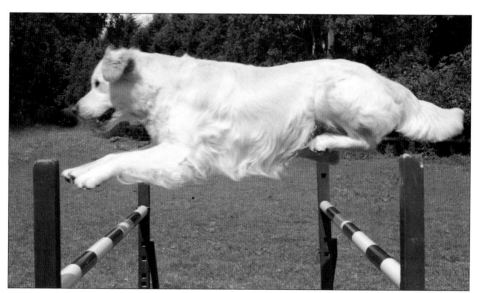

82 The flight. (Courtesy of Henry Robertson.)

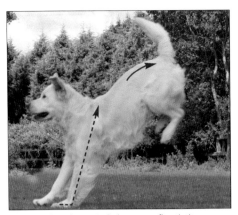

83 The landing. Solid arrow: flexibility; broken arrow: stability/concussion. (Courtesy of Henry Robertson.)

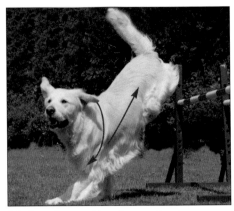

84 Jumping and landing on the transverse plane (rotational). (Courtesy of Henry Robertson.)

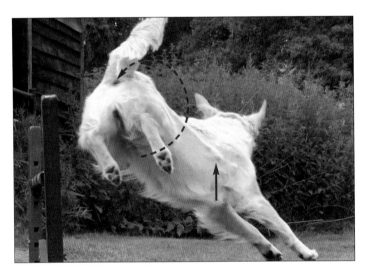

85 Landing and turning immediately; broken line: turning using transverse plane; arrow: landing and twisting off one leg.

On landing, the dog must contend with strong concussive forces in the thoracic limb (83). The full impact is received on the metacarpal pad of one of the thoracic limbs; this is a momentary event when the full weight of the dog is taken by one leg. The landing leg is decided by directional requirement, the mobility and function of the joints, as well as the musculature of each of the legs. Constant use of a particular leg due to musculoskeletal problems will eventually cause a complete lack of function of the region. The shoulder area will receive the impact and softens the landing through its fluid qualities. The dog now readies itself to power into the next stride.

When the dog is asked to land and turn immediately, the requirements are more complex, necessitating the dog to move through a transverse plane (**84, 85**). There is a torque effect on the whole body. The action involves greater impact being received through the landing pad and, more importantly, massively increases the stress running through the m. latissimus dorsi that, if compromised, impacts on the pelvic region. (The reader should refer to fascial planes in Chapter 2.)

Agility

This dynamic sport is completed at speed with many different twists, turns, and obstacles, all in a time-span of about 30 seconds (depending on the course). The activity involves jumping; turning; and running up a 45° incline, stopping, then running down the other side. Fit dogs relish the challenge and enter into the ring with huge amounts of excitement and enthusiasm. Muscles involved in agility are presented in *Table 12*.

With the complexity of movement at speed, training and conditioning are extremely important. The potential for injury is great, and is exacerbated if the injury is unobserved or ignored. Dogs fired with adrenaline and devotion to their handlers will compete when their bodies are injured either acutely or chronically, and will not necessarily employ any self-limiting mechanisms. Furthermore, if dogs were ridden, like horses, we would feel the imbalance; but we instead rely on observation, which is not as reliable, and injuries can be easily ignored.

The likely signs of muscular injury in an agility dog are:

- Reduction of speed.
- Reluctance to enter ring, jump, perform over certain obstacles, or perform contacts.
- Measuring (when a dog approaches a jump in a staccato manner).
- Lack of fluidity when jumping.
- Taking off too close to the jump.
- Taking off too far away from the jump.
- Stiffness/lameness post-event.
- Sensitivity of the foot.
- Lack of coordination when running down an A-frame.

When still photos showing points of impact, movement, or power are studied, it becomes clear why the areas of tension are formed (see **84**). The importance of incorporating the development of postural and core muscles through exercise and training becomes apparent as the figures display how the dog has to move through different planes of movement (see **92**).

Table 12 Muscles and muscle groups involved in agility

Pectorals
Trapezius
Brachiocephalic group
Latissimus dorsi
Supra- and infraspinatus
Carpal flexors
Biceps brachii
Brachialis
Longissimus group (especially lumbar)
Lumbar iliocostal
Hip flexors including the psoas and iliacus
Middle gluteal
Adductor group
Hip extensors including quadriceps group and sartorius
Hamstring

Figure **86** shows the typical areas of stress in the jumping agility dog. Dotted areas indicate pectoral (cranial) and adductor (caudal) muscles. The areas highlighted may seem excessive, but when the range of equipment that is used for agility training is taken into consideration, the reason why becomes more apparent. The main areas of stress are in the shoulder area, especially the thoracic regions of the m. trapezius and m. rhomboideus. These are the areas that receive concussion when landing after a jump (**84**), when twisting through the weaves, and when upholding contacts (a compulsory feature of agility that requires the dog to stop on, or touch with the feet an allocated area of equipment), but not running contacts.

Figures **87** and **88** show a large dog (Jasper) and a small dog (Oscar) negotiating old-sized weaving poles. Jasper is seen negotiating a tunnel in Figures **89** and **90**. The stresses of both tunnel entry and exit for a large dog like Jasper can be seen, and explain the cause of his repetitive lumbar and sacral problems.

The carpal joints are also hyper-extended each time a dog lands from a jump or stops on an incline (**91**). These

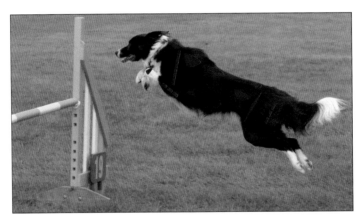

86 Stress areas in the agility dog jumping (on the sagittal plane). Dotted areas indicate pectoral (cranial) and adductor (caudal) muscles. (Courtesy of Henry Robertson.)

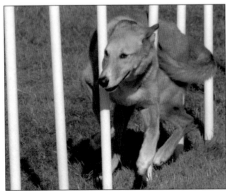

87 Jasper in old-sized weaving poles. (Courtesy of Jay Photos, Cornwall.)

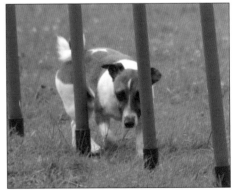

88 Oscar in old-sized weaving poles. (Courtesy of Henry Robertson.)

joints become extremely tight and the retinaculum can start to restrict both flexion and hyperextension through the thixothopic stresses and fascial tension (see **88**). If this is affected, the concussional effect and fascial tension through the shoulder will tighten, causing a reduction of speed, as well as a reluctance to jump and hold contacts. This is further affected by tension of the m. latissimus dorsi caused, in part, by twisting from the sagittal to the transverse plane when landing and turning (**92**). Tension in this muscle can further affect the pelvic alignment.

If a dog does not have the postural support through the coxofemoral joint (primarily due to lacking m. middle gluteal development), the pelvic region will be under additional stress; compensation will be found in the deep lumbar region, causing hypertrophy in the mm. internal and external obliques in an attempt to protect and stabilize the region.

The lumbar region is the other area of issue for the agility dog, especially the deep hip flexors that subsequently shorten through overuse and injury. Ultimately, this impacts on pelvic angulation and

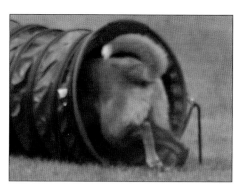
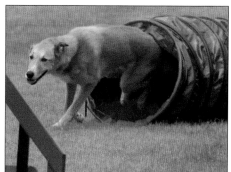

89, 90 Jasper entering and exiting a standard-sized tunnel. (Courtesy of Henry Robertson; reproduced by kind permission of Jasper Bolton and Oscar Norgate.)

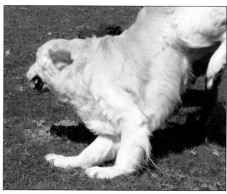
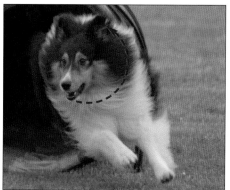

91 Carpal hyperextension on landing.

92 Rotational effect of the turns on the shoulders. (Courtesy of Tony Le Signe.)

causes problems to the sacroiliac joint. An experienced agility dog that has had plenty of training on the flat develops good pelvic stability and uses the hip flexor group appropriately in weaving, using both concentric and eccentric contraction with each weave pole (**93**). If a dog is not taught to develop good lumbar and pelvic support through appropriate exercises, the inclination is for the dog to 'roach' the back (flex at the thoracolumbar junction) rather than to flex the pelvis. This consequently impacts on the deep hip flexors, requiring them to act as stabilizers. This can become evident through heat developing in the mid-thoracic region and a slight roaching effect appearing in the lower back (**94**).

Flyball

Flyball is an unbelievably dynamic and frenzied sport which can be played in slightly different ways, depending on the rules being applied. However, the basic moves are similar. The dog activates the trigger for a ball to be propelled from a box which the dog retrieves by jumping over a line of small hurdles (**95**). Unlike agility, the variation of the moves and planes of movement are not present as often. However, the potential impact from hitting the box at speed, or the spin action needed sometimes for catching the ball, can impact greatly on the whole of the body. The muscles involved in flyball are shown in *Table 13*.

Table 13 Muscles and muscle groups involved in flyball
Pectorals
Trapezius
Brachiocephalic (group)
Latissimus dorsi
Supra and infraspinatus
Carpal flexor
Biceps brachii
Brachialis
Longissimus group (especially lumbar)
Lumbar iliocostal
Psoas and iliacus
Hip flexor
Tensor fascia latae and sartorius
Adductor group
Quadriceps
Hamstring

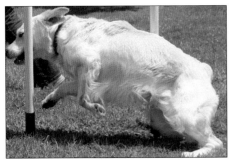

93 An experienced agility dog demonstrating good pelvic stability uses the hip flexor group appropriately, using both concentric and eccentric contraction with each weave pole.

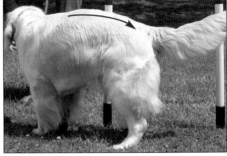

94 An untrained dog will initially 'roach' or flex its back at the thoracolumbar junction (arrow) when going through weaves, without engaging pelvic drive.

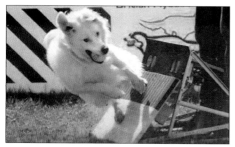

95 Minty playing flyball. (Reproduced by kind permission of Lisa Bishop.)

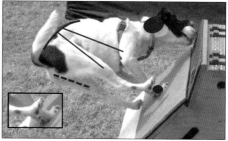

96 Casey playing flyball. Inset shows hyperextension of the carpus. (Reproduced by kind permission of grandimages.biz.)

Figure **96** demonstrates the exaggerated and extreme concussional affects involved in hitting the box. Note the hyperextension of the carpal joint and the flexibility required through the lumbar region. Similar injuries to those of the agility dog are typical through the lumbar region and involving the entire hip flexor group. As always, postural and core strength is crucial, especially through both thoracic and pelvic adductor groups, which support the limbs on the turn. Another key area is within the shoulders; if this area is compromised by poor flexibility and support, the carpal joints will receive more of the concussion. As a result, the recoil action of the carpus will be reduced, which greatly affects the joint congruity. It also impacts on the neck, causing pain when the box is activated.

The typical signs of muscular problems in a flyball dog are:

- Slower times.
- Reluctance to perform.
- Lack of enthusiasm to hit the box.
- Avoidance behaviours.
- Dry nose (see Companion dogs).
- Sensitivity of feet to the touch.

Obedience

The obedience dog is the canine equivalent of the dressage horse. Anyone familiar with dressage will recognize the requirements for fitness and conditioning in order to have the ability and coordination needed to hold the movements required with a fine degree of accuracy. The difference between this type of activity in the dog and horse is that the dog has to hold his head up, putting more strain on his lower back. This is completely different from the afore-mentioned highly dynamic sports of agility and flyball. However, it is equally demanding, and requires the same amount of fitness and conditioning. *Table 14 overleaf* presents the muscles involved in obedience training.

In some respects, this discipline, practised at a high level, is one of the toughest for the dog's musculoskeletal system. The amount of static and eccentric contraction required to hold a position at a slow pace requires a high amount of energy and complete balance control. An example of the type of pressure which is applied to the pelvic region would be that of the classic pre-ski exercise in humans; here, the person stands with their back against a wall, slides down until the knees are flexed and the feet are the same distance away from the wall as the length of the femur, and holds. This is a static contraction of the quadricep group (and other muscles). There is no movement, the body is held still against gravity. When a dog is performing at slow pace and moving through hocks, this is almost what it is doing.

Figure **97** shows angulation of the head with the referred stresses reflecting through the thoracic and lumbar regions, and isolated within the gluteal muscles. Figure **98** shows flexion of the hock and stifle area. Other effects include:

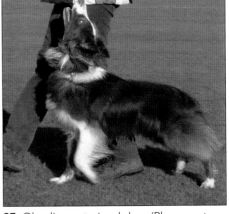

97 Obedience trained dog. (Please note: this head position was freely offered by the dog; it was not forcibly trained.)

Table 14 Muscles and muscle groups involved in obedience training
Pectorals
Trapezius/rhomboideus
Splenius
Psoas/iliacus
Latissimus dorsi
Longissimus group (especially lumbar)
Lumbar iliocostal
Gluteals
Hamstring group
Gastrocnemius
Quadricep group
Tensor fascia latae
Sartorius
Adductor group

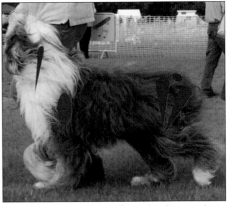

98 The stress points of an obedience dog. Note the flexion of the hock and stifle area. (Courtesy of Henry Robertson.)

- The continual spinal curvature to the right with the head inclined puts huge pressure on the whole vertebral system.
- Reflective stress passes through the body from the neck, and the slight curvature will, in some instances, cause instability thorough the pelvic region (if the lumbar region is long).
- The concentric contraction of the hamstring group during the slow pace will cause stress and overuse problems if dogs are not conditioned and trained appropriately. The obedience dog needs to work using opposite stresses of the vertebrae, both in flexion of the neck, and opposite flexion of the vertebrae.
- The overworking of the hamstring group and the adductors will cause a gradual shortening of these muscles, which will then stretch the quadricep group, and cause the classic 'pelvic slide' if not treated.
- The prolonged eccentric contraction of the gluteal muscle group may cause repetitive strain problems.
- The left shoulder due to continual maintaining of posture and closeness to the handler's leg, and the right shoulder being used as a constant pivot.

The likely signs that an obedience dog has muscular imbalance are:

- Inability to hold a gait.
- Deliberating over stance control.
- Lateral swinging of the pelvic region.
- Reluctance to perform a particular part of a discipline, e.g. not hold a sit.

The risk of a chronic neck injury also means the potential loss of scenting ability, as this has a direct relationship with some neck problems. A key indicator is if the dog has a dry nose (see Chapter 5).

Gundogs

Through training and conformation, the gundog has the advantage of being built

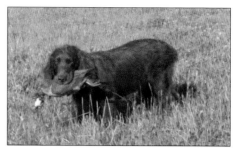

99 Copper, a working gundog.

for the job. However, diverse farming patterns mean that on a 'drive' they could be working on a ploughed field one moment and then on 'set aside' (unfarmed) land the next. The going on these surfaces is very different, so their handlers must be able to supervise them while they are running and possibly carrying their quarry (99).

Due to the diversity of training methods employed and the lack of repetitive actions during the course of their work, the gundog's postural development is generally quite sound. They are more likely to suffer accidents when negotiating obstacles, such as wire fences, stiles, and rabbit holes, but as they may be working out of sight, these incidents may go unnoticed. Because of the type of work and the conditions, these dogs are more likely to suffer from microtrauma, which would not show up on the day, but would be noticed afterwards, as post-shoot day stiffness. This would not necessarily be a major issue, but if left without treatment, the injury could be exacerbated and cause compensatory problems, leading to reduced working ability.

The main area of strain is in the neck (**100**). Sometimes the size of the game can be disproportionately large for the size of the dog. To carry a bird over an uneven field or from water can be an extremely arduous task that takes a huge amount of static muscular force to perform. Although gundogs are bred for the task, the neck is an area that needs attention and can, consequently, cause strain further down the dog's back, especially when it is fatigued, or if it is retrieving over a long distance or over difficult ground. As previously mentioned, a good indication that a dog has an impaired neck is a dry nose (see Chapter 5), which can mean that the dog will not have the same ability to pick up a scent. This is a potential disaster, as the ability to scent is crucial for a gundog.

Another problem area for the gundog that retrieves is that, between the drives, there is opportunity for the dog to get cold. Keeping them warm is key; it may seem excessive for a working dog, but if it keeps warm, it will remain in a state of homeostasis. Consequently, the muscles will provide the movement and stability

required to perform their tasks efficiently, rather than having to keep the dog warm. The dog will also feel more in a state of readiness; its muscles will be more relaxed, and valuable nutritional resources will be available for activity rather than thermo-regulation. This really applies too during break periods, or at the end of the day; keeping the dog warm assists muscle repair and assists free movement to aid fibre realignment.

Another area worthy of note could be on how much road work exercise the gun dog receives both 'on' and 'off' season. The feet are a key stress area that affects many working gun dogs, suffering osteoarthritic changes that can reduce their working life. This may be due to the lack of road working that assists the tightening of the integral tendons within the foot, resulting in a lack of good stability within the joints. As the gun dog covers uneven ground, often carrying a weight (dummy or bird), such changes in joint work load could lead to arthritic changes. A small amount of soft road working, gentle trotting and walking, a couple of times a week for just 10 minutes could help reduce this incidence.

Possible indicators of muscular problems in a working gundog are:

- Post-working stiffness.
- Reluctance to work over difficult or uneven ground.
- Reluctance and difficulty in jumping.
- Lack of speed of the retrieval (dropping and picking up).
- Lack of drive.
- Reduced scenting ability.

Husky sledding

If a Husky has an appropriate harness (**101**), the main pulling effort comes from the sternal region, a central point in the dog, resulting from the dog pushing through the harness. This drives the force from a low point of gravity up through the thoracic region and through to the pelvic region. This route almost exactly follows

100 The most common areas of muscle problems in a gundog.

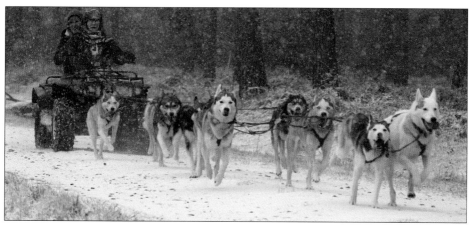

101 Huskies on the way home after exercise. (Courtesy of Henry Robertson; reproduced by kind permission of C. Kisko.)

102 Stress areas in the working Husky. Note also the line of the harness. (Courtesy of Henry Robertson; reproduced by kind permission of C. Kisko.)

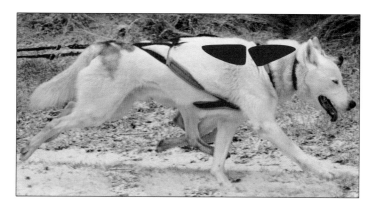

the fascial planes, so the muscles are aided by their tensile strength. This facilitates the pelvic region to drive through the lumbar region, thereby creating an appropriate kinetic chain of forward action and drive.

Figure **102** shows the similarity of the stress lines of the working dog and the anatomical fascial lines. These demonstrate potential problem areas should a dog be constantly put in a position which would cause it to develop stress down one side, especially if paired with a dog of unequal power or stamina. The stresses would differ if an inappropriate harness were used.

Examples of muscular problems in a working Husky are:

• Paddling (at a standstill).
• Running off-line.
• Fatiguing prematurely.
• Slack line (not pulling in line).
• Running off centre line.

Canicross

This is a relatively new sport to the UK, but it is extremely popular in the rest of Europe. It is open to all breeds, and involves both dog and handler running a set course of about 3–5 km in varied terrain, from open fields to forest trails. Some Canicrossers are also covering 10 km to marathon distances, primarily off-road, avoiding concrete, tarmac, and sharp rocky surfaces to protect the dogs' feet and minimize wear and tear of both dog and runner. It is growing in popularity, and is the complete dog and handler combined competition. It involves a dog and its handler being attached by a harness which has been specifically designed for the task. There is no rule that a harness should be worn, but for safety of both dog and handler it is the preferred option. It is desirable for the dog to pull out in front; heeling is acceptable, although this will have an impact on how the dog moves.

The type of harness worn must be considered carefully by the competitor. It must be designed for this use, and not an adaptation of one that was intended for another purpose. An example of this is a harness that has been designed as a sled harness and is intended for a dog 'pulling' with the stress being taken parallel to the object it is fixed to (see **102**). However, in Canicross, the dog will be at an angle to the handler, and the angle will differ with each handler and dog combination. This incorrect angulation could affect the dog's lumbar region. The standard length of connecting line between dog and runner is 2 m at full extension. If, however, a tall person is running with a Jack Russell terrier, then the line must be long enough; otherwise, there would be unnecessary upward pull on the dog. This would impinge on the dog's movements and cause discomfort. In addition, lines are advised to be elasticated to avoid jolting of runners' backs and dogs' shoulders and necks. However, too much elastication could result in whiplash-type injuries for the dog.

It is important that the dog's harness does have a good anchorage point that remains on the manibrium (the cranial part of the sternum) and does not impede the pectoral muscles that lie adjacent to it. It must allow good shoulder movement and also facilitate friction-free movement of the m. latissiumus dorsi. The harness should fit both dog and handler exactly. The handler's harness should also fit well, and it is best if it is put on the lower lumbar/upper pelvic region; this would provide most strength without causing excessive stress on the lumbar or abdominal regions.

Both dog and handler have to be fit for this event, and the stress areas are the same for both (**103**). Everything depends on the terrain, especially the amount of uphill and downhill work involved, as this affects the stresses that would be involved.

Show dogs

A well-muscled dog will attract the judge's eye in its first circuit around the ring. A dog that is balanced and can 'push away' from the hindquarters will set itself apart from the rest. When being presented to the judge, whether freestanding, stacked, or top-and-tailed, a dog that can stand four-square is what is being sought by good judges. If the dog is evenly muscled and balanced, this will be natural. The show dog that has been prepared with correct ring-craft activities will have developed good core stability (**104**). Appropriate exercises encourage core and postural strength so that a dog can show very well, both through the moving and static phases of the competition. Massage to help warm the soft tissue can act as an important tool to demonstrate the dog's full range and ease of movement, as well as acting as a good bonding experience for handler and dog (see Warm-up (pre-event) massage and Warm-down (post- event) massage).

The show dog has no specific problem areas, apart from travelling in crates and lying on benches that do not allow the dog to stretch and move for prolonged periods.

However, if it sustains an injury, even a very small one, this could affect its gait and range of movement, and this could compromise the dog's opportunity to represent its true quality.

Companion dogs

Man's best friend is a very true statement and the role of the companion dog has made a positive difference to many peoples' lives. The companionship cannot be underestimated in its value. Most people want to reward their dogs for their unconditional love; however, unknowingly, we can sometimes present our dogs with environmental complications that can have a devastating effect on their long-term health (**105**).

The companion dog can be affected by many different potential problems, including:

- Extensive weekend walks.
- Inappropriate jumping.
- Excessive ball play.
- Slippery floors.
- Stairs.

Extensive weekend walks

Maybe one of the most problematic dogs is the 'weekend walker'. During the week, this dog is given a 10 minute walk around the block in the morning and the same in the evening. However, at the weekend it is taken on a greatly extended walk lasting many hours. The exuberance shown by the dog is obvious, but the potential for injury is great and can start when the dog is a puppy and not skeletally capable of dealing with this amount of exercise.

This may not be demonstrated as overt injury, as the post-walk stiffness would wear off during the week. A slow somatic change will ensue, however, probably starting in the cervical and shoulder areas, where there will be developing tension throughout the region. This will be caused by jumping down from obstacles and excessive running, and occurs if the dog is too young, or not warmed up.

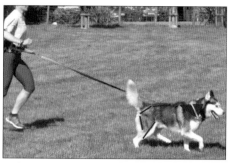

103 Stress points of the dog during Canicross. (Reproduced by kind permisson of Canicross Trailrunnners.)

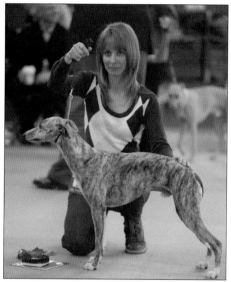

104 Show dog 'Tiggi' and Kerry. (Reproduced with kind permission of BJ Photography.)

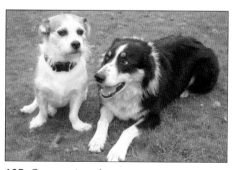

105 Companion dogs.

Inappropriate jumping

Another classic scenario is that of putting the dog in the car to go for a walk. When arriving at the destination and opening the back of the car, the dog leaps out, rushing off from a standing start into a flat-out gallop, or, worse still, being thrown a ball or Frisbee. The impact of both these activities can be clearly seen on photos. It involves going from a 'cold' muscular state straight into a high level of activity, fired by adrenaline, which is not very good for the dog. These repeated actions will lead to minor back and shoulder injuries, which would probably be apparent as some minor stiffness that would occur after any form of exercise, and therefore be disregarded.

This is then worsened by the dog jumping on and off furnishings. These unnoticed injuries can cause scarring of the muscles; this reduces their ability to function properly, and causes them to shorten, putting stress on the joints. The shortening of the muscle will gradually impact on joint congruity and will start

the compensatory process. If the injury is in the back, the dog will compensate and try not to use the drive muscles in the pelvic limbs and pelvis, and will start to power from the front, building and developing these muscles as drive muscles (see Chapter 6 – the torpedo).

In Figures **106** and **107**, the strain jumping down from a car puts on the front region of the dog is evident. This area is designed to absorb this kind of impact; however, when dogs are cold, the recoil and absorption effects of the muscles are compromised. If this occurs frequently, the repetitive action will have an impact on the musculature of the shoulder. The solutions, as mentioned earlier, include using a good ramp or a supporting sling, or lifting the dog in and out of the car if it is small enough. (The author's own dog was used to demonstrate this action and, later that evening, there was distinct heat within the m. trapezius and he was unsound the following day, then fine the day after. He was subsequently treated and the stress issues have been alleviated.)

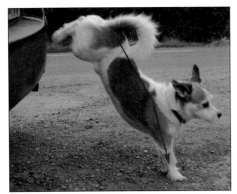 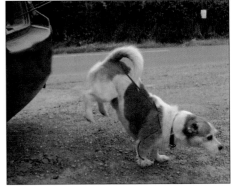

106, 107 The stresses on a dog's body as it jumps out of a car. (Courtesy of Henry Robertson.)

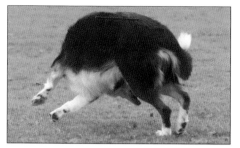 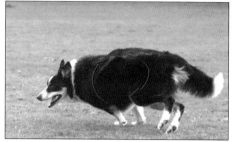

108, 109 Dog chasing a ball. The line in (**108**) indicates the stress of torque through the vertebrae; the arrows in (**109**) indicate the opposing stresses of the rapid turn. (Courtesy of Henry Robertson.)

Excessive ball play

Ball play to a dog represents the chase of a hunt and the subsequent capture of the quarry. The dog has an intrinsic desire to do this, but some types do more than others. However, this can be exploited by excessive ball play – how many rabbits would a dog really hunt and kill in one day, compared to the number of time a ball is thrown? The simple repeated action of chasing a ball creates a massive amount of stress through the torque effect of rotation. If Figures **108** and **109** are studied closely, it is evident that the dog twists in two different directions, causing a huge amount of stress in the vertebral column. If this is repeated over a long period of time, it will cause a large amount of insidious low-grade injury, or more damaging joint disease.

Slippery floors

As far as cleanliness is concerned, laminate, wooden, or tiled floors have a lot to commend them; however, when it comes to a dog's stability when walking or running, the lack of traction can have some extremely long-lasting effects. Dogs' legs can violently hyper-abduct if they are slipping, causing sprains and strains within joints and surrounding soft tissue, causing long-term damage. Also, if the dog already has instability problems, these flooring types can exacerbate them.

Stairs and furniture

Both ascending and descending stairs and jumping on and off furniture can cause the same types of repetitive strain injuries as can jumping in and out of a car. These continual activities are at their most potentially damaging when the dog is very young or adolescent, with an under-developed skeletal system. These continual stresses can have a major impact on both the muscular and skeletal systems. The skeletal system is badly affected by the constant general stress, inappropriate stresses involved in landing, and excessive flexion and extension caused by the propulsion required. These can all damage the growth plates (see Chapter 2). Regarding the muscular system, these movements create microtrauma of the fibres as a result of the propulsive forces required. Thus, concessional muscles are recruited; this will create a change in directional contraction or reduced relaxation within these muscles that will subsequently affect the directional stress on both the skeletal and muscular systems, and therefore cause changes in muscle and joint patterns and congruence to accommodate the traumas.

Warming up and warming down

The subject of warming up and down is contentious, and one that some scientific studies have dismissed as unnecessary. Interestingly, top athletes, whether they are runners or team players, always have warming up period as an essential part their routine. Rugby players are now often seen on static bikes, pitch-side, warming up; racehorses are given the opportunity to run before a race; show jumpers, eventers, and dressage competition horses, are all given a practice area in which to warm up, whatever the level of competition. This is generally viewed to be an essential part of any athlete's programme; unfortunately, there are very few canine shows that involve athleticism, and therefore, the importance of warming up and down is barely considered. Interestingly, the warm-down seems to have more credence and is more widely accepted than the warm-up.

Why warm up?

The warm-up should be a programme of exercises that effectively targets the muscle groups which are to be used. It does not necessarily need to be used just in training, performing, or competition; the concept of a warm-up and warm-down should apply to every exercise situation. It usually consists of dynamic and static elements that will assist the functioning of the soft tissue, so as to maximize the range of movement. It is also psychologically important, as the routine will focus the mind on the task ahead, which is extremely important for a dog.

The physiological benefits of dynamically warming up are, in some cases, open to conjecture. However, any preparatory increase of oxygenation and nutrition from the blood through increased cardiovascular activity is going to promote and prolong muscle function. On a cellular level, if muscle fibres are activated with a moderate approach, the resulting ease of movement is evident.

Therefore, it would be fair to think that the elasticity, stretch, and recoil would all be enhanced. Also, the movement and joint activity of synovial joints will decrease the viscosity of synovial fluid, thereby aiding their smooth function.

The warm-up should take around 10 minutes and consist of gradually increasing cardiorespiratory activities, building up in intensity, speed, and gently progressing movement. Gentle and slow small circling should be introduced, with a gradual increase of circumference, in both directions; tracing out the letter 'M' can then be integrated to encourage an even stretch. Lateral movements can be introduced (adduction and abduction) when the dog is warm. Ball throwing should not be introduced until the dog is completely warm, and this should be restricted to one or two throws. Tugging can be introduced, again when the dog is warm, but this exercise should ideally be restricted to a direct pull, as this helps fire the vertebral postural muscles. Violent shaking of the neck should be restricted.

Warm-up (pre-event) massage

This can be an important addition to a dynamic warm-up, but it is not a replacement.

'The massage techniques l was taught helped prepare my dogs for competition. Particularly at Crufts with Tally, when massaging him in the collecting ring definitely helped us both relax and enhanced the connection between us.'

Tania Bull (see **110**)

The warm-up massage produces both quantifiable and unquantifiable results. When a dog is timed on a regular basis for a round, or its mobility is being measured, fine differences can be accounted for. Chance and coincidence can always be a possibility, but when the same results are achieved with the same preparation, they can be believed. However, there are times when a dog seems more focused, and is

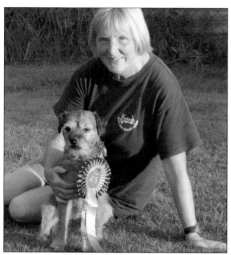

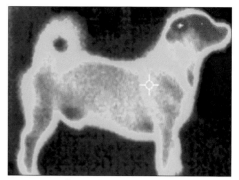

111 Dog after a dynamic warm-up only (lighter areas: cooler; darker areas: warmer).

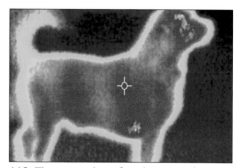

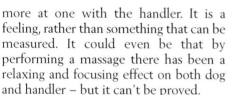

110 Tania and Tally's first time at Crufts in agility – they came second. (Reproduced by kind permission of Steven Bull.)

112 The same dog after the same dynamic warm-up followed by a pre-event massage, photographed 20 minutes later.

more at one with the handler. It is a feeling, rather than something that can be measured. It could even be that by performing a massage there has been a relaxing and focusing effect on both dog and handler – but it can't be proved.

Pre-event massages can be used in different ways for different activities. For instance, the agility dog needs to be stimulated and alert, whereas an obedience dog needs to be more contained and focused. Similarly, a gundog would need to be continually warmed between drives to maintain optimum muscular efficiency and reduce the risk of injury through cold muscles. The rate of the massage can be adjusted accordingly: the quicker the massage, the more stimulatory it is, as the sympathetic nervous system is being influenced. If a more focused disposition is needed for an event, then the rate can be slower. This is also applicable if a pre-event massage is being introduced earlier into the routine.

In an attempt to demonstrate the difference between a dog that has been dynamically warmed and a dog that has been dynamically warmed and then massaged, a heat-sensitive (thermal imaging) camera was used to photograph a dog before (111) and after (112) massage. The massage clearly helped to increase the dog's temperature.

A warm-up or pre-event massage aims to:

- Warm superficial tissues by frictional heat and, therefore, to prepare them for activity.
- Warm deeper soft tissue by influencing arterial circulation providing increased oxygen and nutrients.
- Prepare the dog mentally and physically for activity.
- Connect and focus both dog and handler.

The warm-up or pre-event massage should consist of:

- Effleurage, starting gently and building up slight pressure.
- Petrissage – kneading, compression.
- Cross-fibre techniques.
- Tendon release.
- Tapotment (dependent on the dog).
- Passive movement.

(For explanations of these techniques, see Chapter 6.)

For optimum effect, this massage should be performed between 20 and 40 minutes before an event, working with the dog and gauging the response and respect. If this is incorporated into the whole routine, it will become second nature to both dog and handler, and becomes a good way to prepare, both physically and mentally.

Why warm down?

'Warming down is preparing the muscles for the next event'.

Galen Therapy Centre

If everyone could view a warm-down and see the way that it can greatly influence a dog's performance in the next event, everyone would do it. To perform a correct warm-down should leave the athlete (injury aside) with little or no post-event muscular stiffness and a feeling of well-being.

A warm-down, like a warm-up, should be dynamic and, if possible, aided by a specific massage. Dynamically, it should take the form of active but not too vigorous exercise. It is best described as exercise of an even tempo, a comfortable active walk or light jog, enough to promote the pumping mechanism through muscular activity, but not enough to be oxygen-demanding. Gentle flexion and extension of the vertebrae and the limbs maintains the mobility of the joints if there is tissue damage. This exercise should last for about 10 minutes.

Like the warm-up, the warm-down is looking to promote capillary function and the filling of the muscles with arterial blood, by influencing and aiding venous and lymphatic return. During exercise, a vast amount of metabolic activity occurs within the muscle fibres; with the correct rebalancing of oxygenation within the muscle cells, metabolic wastes will be removed effectively (see Chapter 2). Aiding and promoting arterial circulation will assist the delivery of good levels of oxygen and nutrition to the muscle fibres. It will also help to remove lactic acid and aid the repair of microtrauma; furthermore, it will ease pain perception from microtrauma or minor injury through the realignment of muscle fibres.

Warm-down (post-event) massage

This is an important addition to a dynamic warm-up. It provides the handler with the opportunity to detect even a small injury. Its importance cannot be understated, as many muscular problems in the canine athlete are due to untreated injuries. The major ones are obvious, as the dog may be lame, stiff, or unsound. However, it is the minor injuries that can develop unseen and cause future problems. To massage the dog gently will, to a degree, smooth the nerves endings (see Chapter 6 – gate control theory) and, perhaps more importantly, identify areas of inflammation by the presence of heat.

To gain the most lymphatic return, the massage should be directed towards the main lymphatic nodes, rather than using the long, sweeping strokes of the pre-event massage.

Possibly one of the most underestimated aspects of a post-event massage is the reinforcing of connections between dog and handler. This can make a massive psychological difference to the dog's outlook and memory of the event. If the competition has gone badly, this is often due to handler error; however, the dog will pick up negativity, regarding any problems as being of their own doing. For most dogs, it is a heinous crime to cause a vulnerability to the pack, and they may see the situation this way. Therefore, the one-to-one massage can reinforce the bond between handler and dog. Through eye contact and touch, the dog receives signals that all is well. For a dog to have good memories of a competition, whatever the result, will bode well for subsequent events.

A post-event massage aims to:

- Get hands-on awareness of possible injury.
- Cleanse and re-oxygenate muscle fibres.
- Influence flow of arterial blood to assist with microtrauma repair.
- Realign muscle fibres to help with muscle function.
- Reinforce the connections between dog and handler.

Even if there is no perceptible injury, post-event massage must be performed gently and sympathetically, with the understanding that there could be areas of tenderness and soreness that are almost imperceptible to the handler. Therefore, this massage could consist only of a moderate effleurage with no other techniques involved. The rule is that if there is any question of there being an injury, this should not be performed. If there is a possibility of an injury, or if the dog is clearly lame, then massage should

not be performed, because if there is intra- or intermuscular bleeding, more damage can be done; veterinary assistance must be obtained.

The warm-down (post-event) massage should consist of:

- Hand placement over the dog to isolate areas of heat or inflammation. If there is heat, massage should not be performed of the area and appropriate cold therapy should be applied.
- Gentle effleurage, directing the strokes towards the main areas of lymphatic drainage.
- Depending on the dog's condition, effleurage with slightly increased pressure.
- Compression techniques.
- Effleurage.
- Gentle cross-fibre technique.
- Tendon-release massage.
- Effleurage.
- Passive movement.

(For explanations of these techniques, see Chapter 6.)

Ideally, this should be done not later than 4 hours after exercise. This is not in any way prescriptive, and care must be taken at all times, as areas with fractured or damaged cells can be worsened by inappropriate massage techniques. Like the pre-event massage, to perform this 48 hours later will assist any cellular repair and fibre realignment, and also alert the handler to any persistent inflammation that should receive veterinary advice.

Additional information for handlers of sporting dogs

- If time elapses between classes, events, or drives, another warm-up is required; do not let dogs get cold between disciplines.
- With high impact and dynamic sports, it is a good idea to get someone to film your rounds in order to witness any incident, so that the treatment of any accident or injury can be more targeted.

- Between events, check the muscular balance of your dog through professional therapy and by implementing appropriate exercise regimes, e.g. incorporating rest days with a blend of lead walking, free running, and, possibly, hydrotherapy. Ball throwing, Frisbee throwing, and other high-impact exercise should be minimized.
- Between activity seasons, develop the dog's core strength and stability through correctly designed and assisted canine excercise physiology.
- Also, use massage and passive movement between competition/events and training days, to assist fibre direction and joint congruity.
- Incorporate scenting exercises to encourage a relaxation of the back muscles and gentle flexion of the neck and back vertebrae (see Chapter 5).
- Check your dog's soft tissue, muscle function, and range of movement to minimize the risk of further injury and the development of future compensatory problems.
- Be aware that training sessions tend to be more intensive and have a higher impact than event days.
- Treat areas of heat appropriately, with ice and rest (see Chapter 7).
- Seek professional help for any injury – even if the dog seems to recover, the injury may remain.
- Target areas of stress for treatments.

Warm-up and warm-down for the handler

It is just as important for humans to warm up and warm down as it is for the dog. The body needs to be prepared for physical activity, whether it is a general warm-up or a more specific one for the activity. Especially in the case of agility, with sharp turns, acceleration, and deceleration, the dog and handler need to be well prepared for the stresses which will be placed upon

them. Stretching is always a subject that is open for debate and opinion. However, everyone finds a routine that suits them, and as long as the muscles are warmed dynamically before stretching, then the benefits should always be felt.

Warm-up increases:

- Cardiorespiratory efficiency.
- Blood flow to the active muscles.
- Oxygen transportation and exchange capacity.
- Muscle contraction and relaxation.
- Mental readiness.

Warm-down benefits include:

- Improves flexibility.
- It removes waste products by the bloodstream.
- It minimizes muscular soreness.
- It prevents dizziness or fainting due to blood pooling.

Format of the warm-up and warm-down

The cardiorespiratory portion of the warm-up should last up to 10 minutes at a low-to-moderate intensity, with the warm-down being active but not orientated towards the cardiorespiratory system. This is possibly what one would view as an adequate preparation. However, a complete warm-up and warm-down consists of appropriate stretches as well. The following basic static stretches can be applied.

The static gastrocnemius stretch (113)

- Stand, facing a wall or another stable object, with both arms extended against it.
- Extend one leg backwards about half a metre. The knee should be straight with the heel on the floor.
- Draw in the abdominal muscles (draw the navel inwards).
- Bend the arms and lean forward toward the wall, keeping the rear foot

flat and pointing forward.
- Contract the gluteals and the quadriceps tightly.
- Hold for 20–30 seconds.
- Repeat on the opposite side.

Static kneeling hip flexor stretch (114)
- Kneel with the front and back legs bent at 90° (the kneeling lunge position).

- Draw in the abdominals and place the hands on the hips.
- Slowly, move the body forward until a mild tension is felt in the front of the hip.
- Hold for 20–30 seconds.
- Repeat on the opposite side.

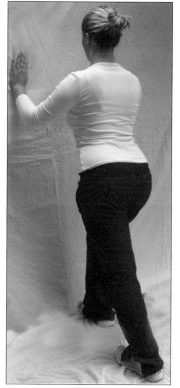

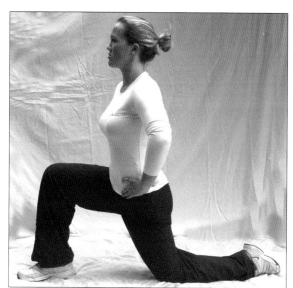

113 Static gastrocnemius stretch.

114 Static kneeling hip flexor stretch.

Static standing adductor stretch (115)

- Stand in a straddled stance with hands on hips; the feet should be further apart than the shoulders.
- Stand with the toes of one foot in line with the arch of the other.
- Draw in the abdominal muscles.
- Slowly transfer weight in a sideways motion towards the leg that is slightly forward until a mild tension in the groin area is felt in the straight leg.
- Hold this stretch for 20–30 seconds.
- Repeat this stretch on the opposite leg.

Static upper trapezius stretch (116)

- Stand with the feet shoulder-width apart.
- Take one arm out to one side of the body in a 45° angle, with the palm facing forward.
- Tuck the chin in and keep the scapula retracted and depressed.
- Slowly move the head in a sideways motion away from the abducted arm (ear to shoulder motion).
- Hold this position for 20–30 seconds.
- Repeat on the opposite side.

Static gluteal stretch (117)

Lie on the back.

- Cross the chosen leg onto the other leg, with the ankle resting just above the knee joint.
- Loop the hands around the thigh of the stabilized leg.
- Pull towards the chest until stretch is felt in the gluteal muscle of the held leg.
- Keep the back and neck aligned (do not aid the stretch with head movement).
- Hold for 20–30 seconds.
- Repeat on the opposite side.

All the stretches shown can be done between events and training to assist muscular function, and can help with repetitive strain conditions. None of these exercises should cause any pain; if they do, stop, and seek medical advice.

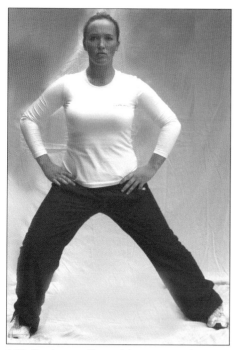

115 Static standing adductor stretch.

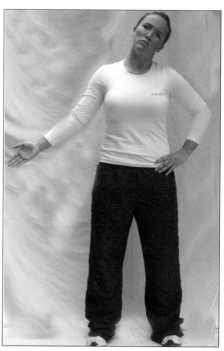

116 Static upper trapezius stretch.

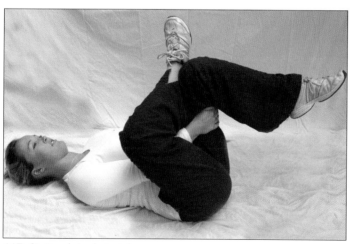

117 Static gluteal stretch.

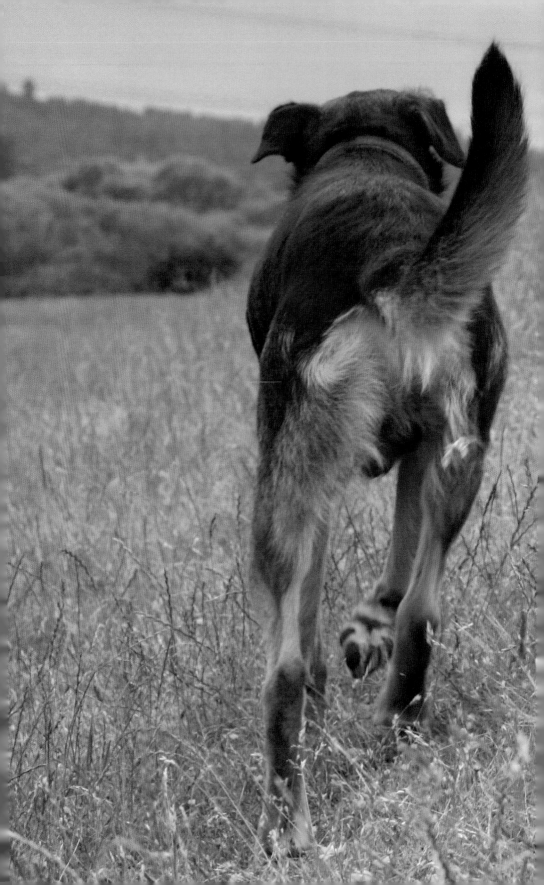

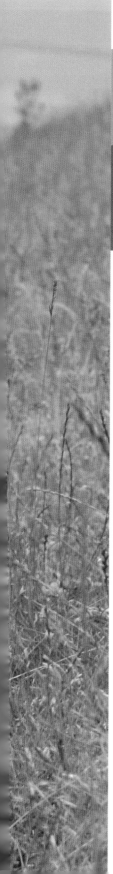

5

Rehabilitation Techniques

Julia Robertson

- Introduction
- Exercising
- Passive movement
- Hydrotherapy

Introduction

In rehabilitation, it is just as important to know what activities to prevent the dog from doing as it is to know what to encourage. Activities such as jumping from cars and the repetitive throwing of balls (see Chapter 4), can reverse the effects of treatment when a dog is recovering from a muscular or joint injury, which may be wrongly interpreted as the treatment being ineffective. This also applies when managing a dog that has a permanent condition, such as osteoarthritis or hip dysplasia. These conditions will deteriorate at a greater rate if such activities are encouraged or not avoided.

The areas covered in this chapter are those that can be safely carried out so as to assist appropriate muscular development and aid mobility following advice from a veterinary surgeon or other specialist. It does not involve the complexity of intricate post-operative physical therapy; however, some areas of post-operative care will be discussed.

Previous chapters have identified areas of stress or overuse within muscles and muscle groups. The exercises that will now be shown will help to repattern the muscles appropriately using simple 'counter-stress' and strengthening techniques that will assist muscle firing, realignment, and resumption of muscle length to regain balance and symmetry. Myotherapy should be integrated regularly within the exercise programme to ensure that the correct muscular patterning is being established, and it should also be part of the timed programme suggested by a therapist to fulfil the realistic expectations for the dog. Also, it is important that these exercises should be demonstrated or explained properly, with a rationale, so that the handler can perform them correctly and understand why they are important.

For the dog that has been, or still is, recumbent, massage, together with some of these dynamic exercises, will help to influence the venous and lymphatic return systems; this will help the dog by replicating exercise and assisting the removal of toxins. This is something that can be easily administered, but one that has many positive effects. The influence on the return systems will cause an enhanced arterial flow that will assist cellular repair and division (see Chapter 2). If applied appropriately, it can soothe and calm a dog that is in pain, and can be especially helpful if the dog is unable to tolerate nonsteroidal anti-inflammatory drugs (NSAIDs). As well as an enhanced circulatory response, massage and passive movement will help a dog neurologically, to regain proprioception and re-establish neural pathways.

When a dog is rehabilitating, especially post-operatively, areas which are distal to those directly affected are also prone to having problems, due to the displacement of weight and change of gait. Massage can be especially helpful in these situations (see Chapter 7).

Exercising

A simple adjustment or adaptation of usual methods of exercise can make dramatic changes to the muscular and joint health of a dog. A straightforward 10 minute lead walk before a longer walk can ensure that the dog is warmed up before running. Then the same 10 minute walk before going home can assist a warm-down. Other exercises that have been prescribed can sometimes be a little difficult to understand, given the circumstances, e.g. post-operatively, post-injury, or post-treatment. These fundamental exercises are relatively easy to adapt, and can make huge differences for the remedial dog.

Lead walking

Lead walking is a vital method of reintroducing or restricting exercise for the dog. It is probably one of the least understood and, therefore, inappropriately performed of all the rehabilitation exercises.

It has different uses for different situations:

- Post-operatively: depending on the operation, it would generally be used to mobilize and promote movement to aid healing and begin to regain the joint's range of movement. The post-operative recumbent dog will regain mobility far quicker if appropriate exercise is introduced into the routine.
- Post-treatment: this would be to contain the otherwise lively dog to obtain the optimum changes from the treatment. To bring about a controlled gait allows muscles to pattern in an appropriate manner without the stress of overexertion. This is generally given a timescale according to the dog's age, condition, normal activity levels, and the treatment received.
- General management of a condition: the amount of lead-walking would depend on the condition; it is used to ease the strain on areas of damage and encourage strengthening of functional regions.

The type of lead used would be dependent on the dog being exercised. If it were an active dog, then a harness would be advisable, to avoid any stresses to the vertebrae that a collar and lead may cause. The only problem with a strong or active dog and the use of a harness can be that of control, as a dog could potentially drag the handler into a potentially dangerous situation. By way of a compromise, the addition of a passive collar and lead, as well as the main lead, can be used. Therefore, if an emergency did occur, the collar can add to the restraining capabilities of the harness. Only in specific cases would lead walking include an extension lead. These leads are intended to allow limited freedom; however, they can produce a catapulting effect as the dog suddenly comes to the end of the lead, and this would be totally counterproductive to any rehabilitation programme.

The type of surface for walking would have to be flat and smooth, as any form of irregularity in the surface would exacerbate a lack of balance. A flat and smooth surface would take out any extra stresses and encourage a regular and smooth gait.

The handler's pace should be adapted to that of the dog, not vice versa, especially if the exercise is for remedial purposes, and the dog encouraged to walk on both sides

Walking

One of the most underestimated rehabilitation exercises is the walk. This is different from the jog or trot as it is 'four time', meaning each leg touches and pushes off from the ground independently. If a dog is encouraged to 'walk', not jog, it will aid rehabilitation and encourage enhanced muscular stability and strength through low impact. A walk can be performed 'slowly' enhancing suspension of movement, therefore encouraging stability, or normal pace, encouraging balance and 'even' weightbearing and use. Extended walk is excellent for helping extension and improved length of stride. The normal and active or extended walk are also excellent inclusions into a warming up routine.

Lateral hill walking

Lateral hill walking (118) can be an extremely efficacious way to develop postural vertebral muscles. Walking along the side of a hill can instigate the use of the crucial muscles that support the vertebrae. It can also be applied to normal strengthening programmes or to remedial programmes where muscle tone has been lost or reduced in the area. This should not be done on very steep hills, but on a gentle gradient. The rationale for these effects is basic, but they can bring about a good response.

Walking the dog slowly and accurately along the side of a hill will encourage the dog to balance through the vertebrae, by contracting the muscles on the higher side concentrically; conversely, the muscle groups on the downhill side will be in

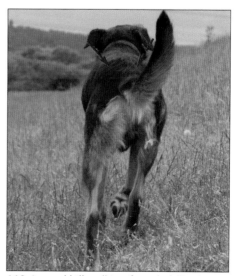

118 Lateral hill walking for rehabilitation. Eccentric contraction: arrow; Concentric contraction: dotted arrow

eccentric contraction, supporting the vertebrae. By changing direction, the muscles of the opposite side of the back will be uppermost, contracting concentrically, while the lower ones are now contracting eccentrically.

Incorporating a gentle turn will also encourage slight lateral movement.

Scenting exercises

Scenting could be one of the most unexploited exercises used with dogs. To set a dog exercises where the nose is encouraged to move toward the ground can help in many different ways. This is a natural position for a dog, and to use this as a form of physical therapy is generally easy to do.

These exercises ease tension within the vertebral column and the shoulders. By putting its nose to the ground, a dog stretches the nuchal ligament and the longitudinal bands of its extension along the back, the supraspinous ligament (see **65**). This is especially useful for obedience dogs, as it is part of their discipline to do much close heel work, which can lead to neck and back problems because of the ventral force created. Indeed, for any dog with shoulder or lower back problems, this is a gentle and natural way to encourage it to stretch out and mobilize the whole vertebral column.

In Figure **119**, the supraspinous ligament is drawn as a solid line. The nuchal ligament (a broken line) is positioned just dorsal to the m. multifidus cervicis. It starts at the spine of the axis and continues caudally to the apex of the first thoracic spine. The supraspinous ligament connects to the apex of the spinous processes of all of the thoracic, lumbar, and sacral vertebrae, and ends at the third caudal vertebra (see also Chapter 3).

This exercise can have highly beneficial effects from a physiological, physical, and psychological perspective. Involving a dog in a game or exercise of scenting will generally have a highly stimulating effect, which will occupy and amuse it by

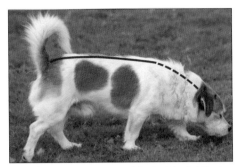

119 Scenting exercise. Nuchal (solid line) and supraspinous (broken line) ligaments.

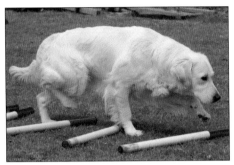

120 Pole walking in rehabilitation. (Courtesy of Henry Robertson.)

engaging one of its greatest senses. By doing this, the dog's mind will be stimulated more than with an ordinary exercise. Therefore, for dogs on a restricted exercise regime, a game of finding small treats, toys, or even its meals, can be extremely satisfying and fulfilling.

Pole walking

Pole walking (**120**) should be incorporated into the routines of puppies and dogs with proprioceptive problems. A couple of poles (up to four) are placed on the ground at irregular spaces; the dog then has to concentrate carefully, choosing which leg to lift to walk over the next pole. This helps to re-establish and develop the neural pathways that constitute spatial awareness and coordination. The more irregularly the poles are placed, the more complex the exercise will be, especially if they are placed at slightly different heights. This causes the dog to concentrate on both distance and height for all four of its legs.

This exercise must be carried out very slowly, with the dog's head down and with its body weight moving forward. If the dog is allowed to walk quickly over the poles with its head up, the rationale will be lost and no gain will be made. The point of this exercise is to encourage the deep supporting muscles to 'fire' or be innervated and, by this, facilitate the dog to use its hip flexors and extensors correctly. Therefore, to get these stabilizing muscles to work, they must be gently encouraged to exert; this exercise, done correctly, will assist this. The exercise can be carried out in a wooded area where there are broken twigs in an irregular format and the dog can walk slowly between and over them. Pole walking should only be done at a walk, with someone attending, especially if it is happening in an uncontrolled environment, e.g. woodland, as the dog must be kept calm and walk at an even pace throughout. This exercise is best performed with expert assistance; if executed correctly it will have huge benefit. However, it is very tiring for the dog and should only be used two or three times per day.

In Figure **120**, note how the dog is aware of where his four feet are in relation to where the irregular poles are lying. Also note the height of the feet and the ease with which it is executing this task. This dog is engaging the correct muscle pattern, enabling balance and ease of extension and flexion to result.

Lateral and medial movements

These exercises (**121**) are extremely good for developing the frontal plane rather than just the sagittal plane. It encourages a dog to walk laterally and medially so that it adducts and abducts both pelvic and thoracic limbs, which helps to develop these groups of muscles that are also important for general postural stability. (These movements are not easy to incorporate in the exercise routine of a dog that is lacking mobility.) It involves getting a dog to walk away from your leg in a sideways manner so that it is, in effect, crossing its legs while walking. Another method is to walk alongside the poles, or their equivalent, used in the previous exercise, and encourage the dog to step sideways over them.

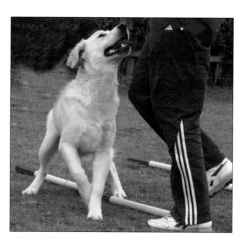

121 Sideways walking over poles (abduction of the pelvic limbs and adduction of the thoracic limbs). (Courtesy of Henry Robertson.)

These exercises can be carefully extended to involve the dog walking alongside a low kerb and with gentle encouragement to step slowly sideways onto the raised surface. This must only be attempted when the dog is confident about stepping over poles laid on the ground.

Stretching

There is much discussion and literature about canine remedial stretching exercises. This is an area that needs careful and precise knowledge, and should not be performed in the general physical therapy arena. Some of the stretches used, in the hands of the untrained, are potentially hazardous to the dog's health. This is because it is possible to manipulate a dog's joint beyond its natural range or mobility, unlike that of a person or horse, whose personal strength and reflex reaction will outmanoeuvre those of the stretcher. This is not to say that stretching is not an important part of physical therapy and massage; it is, and the uses within remedial care are manifold. But it should only be performed by someone with excellent anatomical and physiological knowledge, and it should have correct directional application.

Passive movement

Passive movement is different from a stretch because it is a movement that is taken up to its natural 'end feel'. If the joint is compromised in some way, the same applies. Passive movement is a highly influential technique and one that is not discussed as much as stretching, possibly because of the simple reason that the name does not conjure up a meaning symbolic of dramatic change as that of a 'stretch'. To integrate passive movement exercise will assist with mobilization from a physical and neurological perspective:

- Physical benefit: passive movement involves managing the balance of muscle and scar tissue. Scar tissue can be the most effective method of maintaining mobility, especially in the case of femoral head and neck excision, where the femur is secured in place by the post-operative scar tissue. This has to be managed so that it can facilitate as close to full range of the limb as possible, and yet maintains stability. During this process, the hip flexor and/or extensors will develop areas of tension within normal muscle tissue; therefore, these two must be balanced and treated accordingly.
- Neurological benefit: it can also assist the re-establishment of neural pathways and influence the Golgi tendon receptors (see Chapter 2) to accept an improved range of movement by relaxing the antagonist; this also reduces the pain cycle.

For the recumbent dog, or one with limited mobility, it is best to perform passive movement with the dog lying on its side. This is important, as if it were standing, to lift one leg of its already unbalanced body could cause it to fall. Flexion and extension movements are the same as in Chapter 6, but with the dog on its side (**122, 123**).

- Passive movement must not be executed by an open wound, on a freshly injured site, on any swollen joint, or to a locked joint.
- The dog must be comfortable and stable – either standing or lying.
- All the moving limbs must be supported above and below the joints.
- It is very important that the joints and tissues have been sufficiently pre-warmed by effleurage.
- Passive movement involves taking the joint through its natural anatomical range of movement – it is not a stretch.
- The passive movement should be conducted slowly so that all the tissues involved have time to adjust without any sudden or erratic

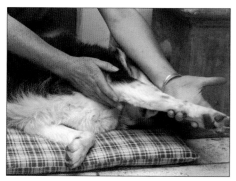

122 Extension of the thoracic limb.

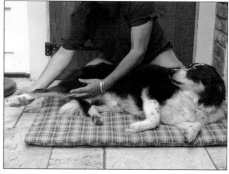

123 Extension of the pelvic limb.

movement; if a joint is moved quickly, damage to the muscle and joint can be inflicted.

- The joint should be held in position (flexed or extended) for at least 15 seconds.
- After every movement, the limb is taken back to a neutral point and held there before the next one.
- Usually three passive moves for each joint are sufficient.
- After passive movement exercises, effleurage or light exercise is used to re-adjust joints and tissues.

Passive movement can also be applied to the neck region. Muscular neck problems in dogs can go unnoticed and, as previously mentioned, a good indicator of a problem can be that of a dry nose. Before any neck movement is attempted, there must be utmost care to ensure that there are no underlying serious neck conditions, such as any spinal damage or disease. This must be checked by a veterinary surgeon.

Extension and flexion of the neck can aid mobility and gently assist the realignment of muscles if it is done along with deep tissue treatments. When performing these exercises be aware that even though they appear to be specific for the neck, they also engage the shoulders and back. Thus, if a dog has back or shoulder problems, these 'neck' exercises can potentially impact on these areas. For this reason, these exercises must be performed sympathetically and with recognition that any restriction could mean a further issue distal to the neck. If at any time a dog is highly resistant to these exercises the dog should be referred for veterinary investigation. Any exercise that involves neck movement must be performed with the greatest care and attention to the individual dog's limits.

An effective neck exercise involves the dog sitting facing the handler, with the neck and head in a forward position in line with the dog's horizontal plane. (This must be especially encouraged in small breeds as the dog is inclined to look up at the handler, drawing the neck into the shoulders.)

- The handler takes approximately four steps backwards with the dog continuing to sit and look directly at the handler. The dog should be sitting as squarely as possible, with their tail directly behind them (**124**).
- The handler then walks in an arc clockwise, from 'half past' to 'twenty to', holding the dog's gaze for 10–15 seconds (**125**). If the dog cannot hold the gaze, or shuffles its feet, the handler moves back to where the dog can comfortably hold the position and resumes timing.
- The handler then returns to the starting position in front of the dog, again encouraging the dog to extend the neck forwards away from the shoulders.
- The exercise is then repeated, but walking to the 'twenty past' position, and is conducted as before (**126**).

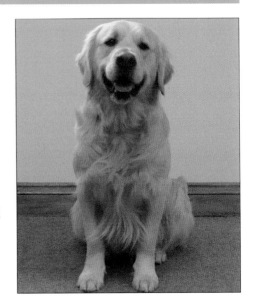

The dog's head should be moving on the horizontal the first time; the exercise can then be repeated with the dog slightly angling its head up and down, but should always be encouraged to extend the neck. In this way, different muscles of the neck and shoulder will be mobilized and softly stretched by the dog. This exercise is highly effective for any dog with neck issues and for general maintenance of range and function. As it involves no intervention from the handler, the dog will only take the extension or flexion to their own range.

To encourage good extension, hyper-extension and flexion exercises (head moving up and down) the following exercise should be conducted, starting with the dog in the same position as in the previous exercise.

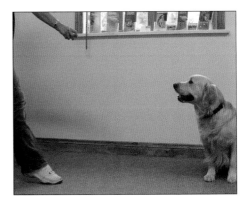

- The handler stands approximately two strides back from the dog.
- Holding their hand on the horizontal to dog's head, the handler encourages the dog to elongate their neck and hold this position for 10–15 seconds.

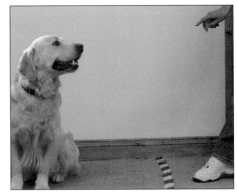

124–126 Flexion and extension of the neck. With kind permission of Galen Natural Progression ©.

- The dog is then allowed to relax, but still encouraging a gentle elongation the handler starts moving their hand in the shape of an arc or through a clock face dimension, starting at 'quarter past' (in line with the dog's nose), slowly lifting their hand upwards and forwards towards '12 o'clock' but stopping just before ('five minutes to the hour').
- The position is held for 10–15 seconds if the dog is comfortable and not shuffling or tilting his head to one side or the other.
- The handler's hand is drawn down encouraging the dog to watch, and stops at 'quarter past' (the start point), again encouraging the dog to elongate their neck.
- The handler's hand moves down towards the floor, again following the line of an arc or clock face, stopping just before' half past'.
- This position is held for 10–15 seconds – remember this will encourage a deep stretch through the caudal border of the shoulders and into the thoracic region.
- The exercise finishes by resuming the start position.

This soft exercise could be repeated once a day in acute and chronic cases. If the dog shuffles his feet, licks his lips, or starts to look away, it could be the handler is asking too much movement for the dog's comfort, so the exercise should demand less movement.

Balance cushion

This form of exercise can be extremely beneficial if applied correctly, after the appropriate therapy. However, the author does not promote the use of many other types of balance apparatus intended for human use, e.g. the Swiss ball. This balance cushion (**127**) allows the dog to demonstrate discomfort easily, giving clear indications of pain that would contraindicate its continued use. The use of the balance cushion for conditions involving pelvic and shoulder instability is highly effective, if used at the correct time. For optimum gain, the dog should only receive treatment which is appropriate to the cushion. Conditions like hip dysplasia can respond positively to this, but only in conjunction with professional therapy.

The aim of this form of therapy is the stimulation of the deep postural muscles of the pelvic or shoulder region. These muscles, in the course of normal movement, may not be neurologically stimulated and, therefore, not involved within movement patterns. To stimulate these using a balance cushion can help to develop good core and postural balance.

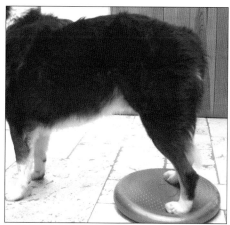

127 A dog standing with the pelvic limbs on a balance cushion.

The idea of the use of the balance cushion is that the weaker muscles will be stimulated rather than the stronger ones; therefore, an equal balance can be achieved if the cushion is used correctly. Like all deep core exercises, this does not give the impression of working muscles hard. However, these small muscles that are being stimulated are having a full workout; care is needed, as if time limits are exceeded, post-exercise hypertonia can be a problem. It is important to ensure that the dog stands as squarely on the cushion as possible. In Figure **127**, note how the right leg is not weightbearing. As this is the stronger leg, the exercise should strengthen the core muscles on the left side. When performing this exercise, the dog should be eased gently so that the opposite pelvic limb is weightbearing (**128**). This, then, should encourage a correction within the intrinsic pelvic muscles.

This exercise should not be performed for longer than 1 minute at the start, and increased daily up to 3 minutes. When the dog can stand squarely, the exercise should be used for maintenance once a week for 3 minutes. This technique should always be replicated with the front legs.

Affected areas (muscles or muscle groups):

- m. gemelli.
- m. obturator internus.
- abdominals.
- obliques.
- m. multidifus.
- gluteal group.

Hydrotherapy

Hydrotherapy is a wonderful tool within the remedial and fitness programme for a dog. For the dog that is paralysed or severely lacking mobility, to have unimpaired movement while supported by water is a great feeling. Not only is hydrotherapy of great benefit to dogs that need to regain mobility, but also there is a social aspect: they may swim with other

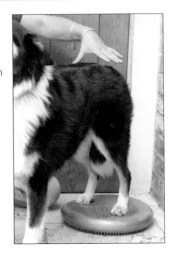

128 The dog is gently moved from the weight-bearing leg to the opposite pelvic limb.

dogs, and the competition can assist a more motivated swim, or give a dog the confidence to swim (**129**). This psychological benefit can be far reaching, and in itself have a wonderful cathartic effect.

In the author's experience, in many chronic and some muscular conditions, to gain best overall results it is advantageous to treat with good myotherapy initially, to rebalance the musculature, thus initiating corrective muscle patterning before a dog engages in hydrotherapy. Hydrotherapy can possibly overdevelop problem areas rather than develop a better overall biomechanical action; in this circumstance, the appropriate use of buoyancy aids adds to the benefit.

If managed correctly and used along with other therapies, hydrotherapy can manifest great changes in a dog's quality of life. From a therapist's perspective, the best results are achieved when the two therapies and therapists can work together. Exercises and massage can ensure that the muscles are released and functioning, so that, when the dog is worked resistively in the water, the range of movement and core muscle strength can be improved.

Before engaging in hydrotherapy, the following should be addressed:

- What is hoped to be achieved by hydrotherapy?
- Which type of pool would be best (**130**)?
- Should another therapy be implemented first?
- How many dogs will be in the pool at the same time (no more than four)?
- What type of dogs will be sharing the pool? Will they be bumptious or placid – which would suit each dog?

- What help would be available should the therapist require it?

The hydrotherapists at these pools may not swim with the dog. Therefore, if specialized care is required when the dog is swimming, a more one-to-one arrangement may be required. Veterinary advice should always be taken before making a decision on which pool the dog swims. Legally, veterinary consent should be required by the hydrotherapist. The subject of hydrotherapy within canine physical therapy is complex and detailed.

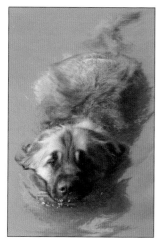

129 Archie swimming in a hydrotherapy pool.

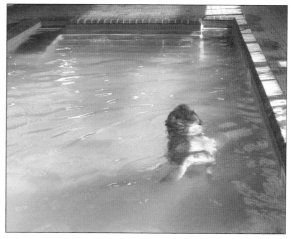

130 A canine hydrotherapy pool; it should have a ramp and steps for entering and leaving the pool and be open to allow the dog to swim freely. (Reproduced by kind permission of White Orchid Hydrotherapy, West Chiltington, Sussex.)

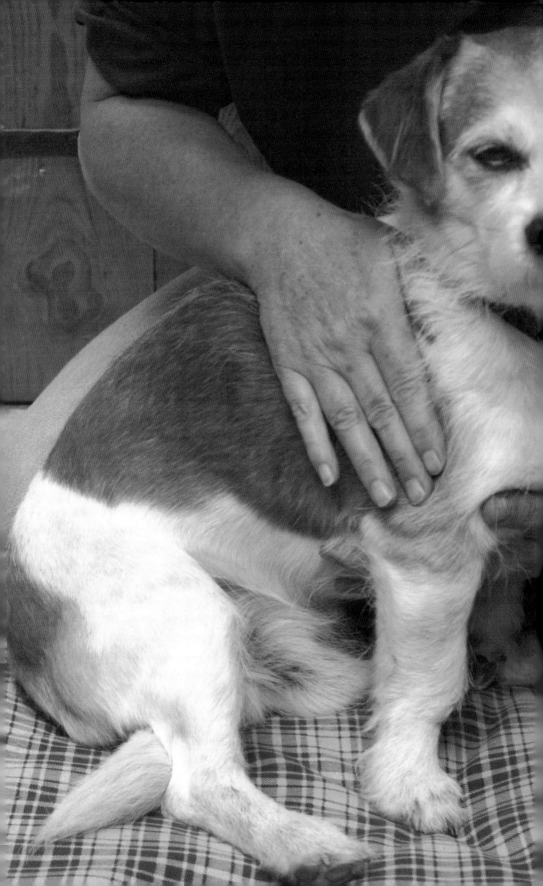

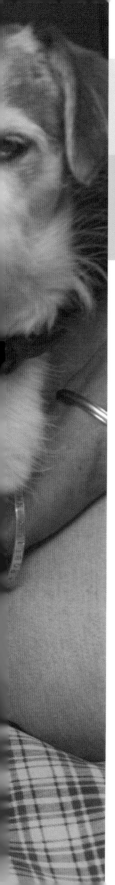

6

Massage in Physical Therapy

Julia Robertson

- Introduction to massage
- Massage methodology
- Massage application
- Massage techniques
- Assessment of the dog
- Treatment
- Contraindications for canine massage

'Society's taboos about touch have kept massage from enjoying the popularity it deserves.'

Dr Michael Fox, The Healing Touch.

'Massage is a manipulation of soft tissue structures of the body. It has both mechanical and reflex effects on the body. The direct form of massage affects the tissues and organs you are working on and the indirect is the reception of a stimulus that produces an effect'.

Beard's Massage. Principles and Practice of Soft Tissue Manipulation. Saunders Elsevier.

Introduction to massage

Massage must never be confused with a therapy that can be mastered easily by reading a book or watching a film. It is an art that has to be practised repeatedly to achieve the appropriate reactions that will facilitate the positive changes that enable the body's healing mechanisms to function, whether human or canine. As with many therapies, especially touch therapies, it has not been entirely substantiated scientifically, but the effects of well-executed treatments cannot all be coincidental. However, it is agreed that our bodily systems interlink. Thus, with the interlinkage and interdependency accepted, the holistic approach connected with this form of treatment cannot be without some firm foundation. For those whose dogs have received treatment and those who have witnessed amazing changes as a result, science does not have all the answers. The changes, both felt and seen, make it difficult to understand why there are still some sceptics who dispute its value; however, any therapy is only as good as the therapist and its appropriateness for the recipient. Massage is generally perceived to be of little use, since its application and effects are not fully understood; however, this can be a potentially hazardous presumption. It is also not considered by many to be as 'serious' as physiotherapy. This is a shame, as the information acquired through the tactile approach used by massage therapists can give a very full picture of past events and injuries. It can also offer an excellent insight into the whole muscular condition of the dog. Unfortunately, it has suffered under the misrepresentation of its history, so many of its benefits have been lost.

Observation is invaluable to a good practitioner. It is extraordinary that Western therapists do not generally consider hair texture, skin feel, and smell to be as important and informative as visual appearance. Good farmers, who have great skills of animal husbandry, learn to use many of their senses to anticipate problems during, for example, calving and lambing. The use of smell is one that can give many clues as to the condition or timing of events; for example, the smell of impending death is not easily forgotten. The body exudes odours from many places. Illnesses can result in a changed odour either through the skin, the breath, or, even in dogs, the feet. Likewise, body or skin condition is reflected through the coat, giving an overall impression of wellbeing or a lack of wellbeing. Thus, an abnormal coat, either partial or total, can indicate an underlying health problem affecting, for example, the neural or circulatory systems.

Observation of behaviour is also critical to the assessment of health. Stretching is an example of this: if a dog gets up after rest and stretches shortly afterwards, this is regarded as a natural and normal healthy response. However, if this action is uneven, e.g. if only the front end or only the hindquarters stretch, this could signify an underlying problem.

Touch is also quite often underestimated as a healing tool. We are all aware of the importance of contact during any young animal's development, but this does not stop at maturity. Touch therapy and massage has proven benefits for both therapist and patient, causing a lowering of the heart rate, and this can lead to reduced stress levels and a reduction of pain perception. This can be explained scientifically by the body's release of endorphins and enkephalins, which are naturally produced chemicals that resemble opiates.

'Massage' encompasses a vast array of therapies, some of which have been patented and named after a particular practitioner. Most appear to date back to early styles of massage and their derivatives. Some concentrate on specific areas of treatment, while others are more general. All of them take practice to perform correctly and to avoid causing damage to the tissue being treated, thereby exacerbating the original problem. There are a myriad of newer therapies available now; it is important to have an understanding of what they are supposed to do, and how. Their names and application methods vary from textbook to textbook. This uncertainty makes the case for having good tactile and palpation skills all the more important.

Massage methodology

Trigger point massage

This is also known as neuromuscular technique. The name 'trigger point' was coined by Dr Janet Travel in 1942.

When a muscle is injured or overused, it lays down fibrous scar tissue, usually within the belly of the muscle/s. This can feel like a nodule and is extremely painful upon palpation. Trigger points are the name given to the centre of the muscular damage, but they refer pain elsewhere in the body along neural pathways. In trigger point therapy, pressure is applied using a thumb or finger directly over the point of damage, the 'trigger point'. Working directly over this point of the muscle that is ischaemic (has a poor blood supply due to its fibrous quality) puts pressure on the area, further restricting the flow of blood. It has a double effect: firstly, on the trigger point and, secondly, on the rest of the affected muscle:

- It draws attention to the point of pain, rather than to the referred pain. This concentrates the neural system in a targeted manner to the 'trigger point' and area of issue. Due to the tension of the affected area and the abnormality within the muscle's fibres, it will have become hypertonic. By relaying a neural alert through the pressure of the digit onto the point of pain and exact point of dysfunction, this can help to facilitate muscle release. This is reinforced by further treatment and correct rehabilitation. The amount and length of pressure exerted by the therapist needs to be carefully managed, as too much pressure is not only extremely painful for the dog, but also can inflict damage to the underlying tissues.
- It also reduces blood flow to the area and triggers a reflexive response, when the pressure is released, directing more arterial blood to the area, and thus facilitating healing.

Interestingly, even though the therapist applies pressure in a manner that creates pain in one area, the body seems to be able to recognize that this is where the referred pain is originating, and can accept the treatment. When treating a dog using this method, if it is executed correctly, the dog's breathing becomes deeper and it relaxes; it seems to become almost entranced until the tension in the area reduces. Simultaneously, it stirs and resumes previous behaviours. This technique must be used only after all the tissues have been warmed and prepared, and mechanical drainage techniques must also be applied to the area, to soothe the nerve endings.

Stress point massage

A stress point is where a mechanical, isotonic force has been so great that it has caused a microtearing of muscle fibres. This tends to happen close to the point of origin of the affected muscles, as this is the anchor point, where most force is reflected. The affected muscles then feel hardened and are tender to the touch. This works very much in the same way as trigger point therapy. By 'triggering' a problem point, it stimulates the natural healing properties that seem to be absent in fibrous and damaged tissue. These stress points are invariably predetermined.

TTouch®

The 'Tellington Touch', after Linda Tellington-Jones, is an awakening of inactive neural pathways and cellular 'intelligence'. This is done by performing circular movements, lifts, and slides over most of the dog's body. Most of what we do and how we move involves a limited pattern of cellular activity. With the rigours of time and minor or major injury, these pathways become restricted and blocked; by awakening these cells, previous behaviours and movements can resume. TTouch also encompasses dynamic exercises and body wraps that are intended to draw the dog's attention to its whole body. Through gentle stimulation, cellular function is awakened and the body is motivated to function correctly, demonstrating natural healing, coping habits, and behaviour. As this treatment is said to be a 'complete therapy', the learning of anatomy and physiology is said to be unnecessary.

Bowen technique

The Bowen technique involves a gentle, rolling motion, with very light touches involving the skin and superficial structures. This causes stretching and heightening sensory awareness of the body in the area where the technique is applied. A treatment session frequently results in a deep sense of relaxation, allowing the body to recharge and balance itself. It stimulates proprioceptors and stretches reflex centres, such as the Golgi tendon organs, eliciting a reflex response. The practitioner stimulates sets of points, then often pauses to allow the body to compute neurologically what has been stimulated.

Connective tissue massage (Rolfing)

This treatment concentrates on influencing the underlying bands of connective tissue called fascia (see Chapter 2). Ida Rolf identified that fascia seemed to adopt different biochemical states according to its state of health. In a state of low hydration, the fascia can become shortened, and it adheres to surrounding tissues, feeling thick and dense to the touch. By manipulating the myofascial bands both locally and more extensively to stimulate cellular change, this treatment enables a correction to develop within cellular lines, and, therefore, creates more balance within these immensely strong and robust bands. This induces an overall neural and physical equilibrium.

Acupressure

Acupressure is often combined with other therapies to work on many levels, including dietary therapy, massage, exercise, meditation, and herbal medicine. It is based on the ancient theories of traditional Chinese medicine (TCM) that have supported the health and wellbeing of animals for over 4,000 years. Some of these theories include Yin-Yang Theory, Meridian Theory, Five Phases of Transformation, and others that help to distinguish specific patterns or conditions. The basic concept of Chi (also seen as QI, or Ki), which underlies TCM, can be described as 'vital life-force energy' that flows throughout the human or dog body. When Chi flows harmoniously, the dog will experience physical and emotional good health. When there is any interruption in the flow of Chi, the dog may experience poor health. Case work has shown that acupressure (131), like acupuncture, can:

- Build up the immune system.
- Strengthen muscles, tendons, joints, and bones.
- Release natural cortisone to reduce swelling and inflammation.
- Release endorphins which increase energy or relieve pain.
- Enhance the mental clarity and the calm required for focus in training and performance.

• Repair injuries more readily, by increasing the blood supply and removing toxins.

The raison d'être of massage is to facilitate change within the body that will elicit healing; this means that a clear understanding of anatomy and physiology is paramount. The two types of technique used are mechanical and reflexive:

• Mechanical: the tissue is physically manipulated so as to aid drainage and increase fluid movement and cellular exchange.

• Reflexive: the reflex actions of the neural and endocrine system are incorporated; for example, proprioception is enhanced or endorphin release is stimulated.

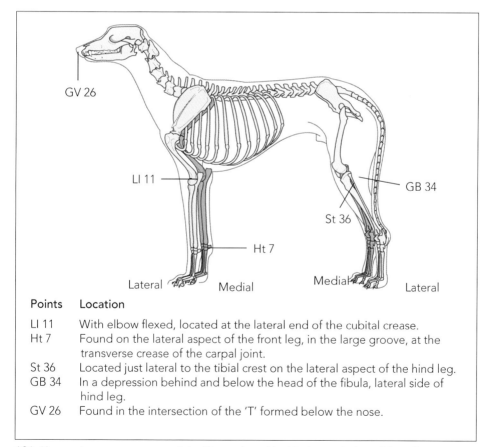

Points	Location
LI 11	With elbow flexed, located at the lateral end of the cubital crease.
Ht 7	Found on the lateral aspect of the front leg, in the large groove, at the transverse crease of the carpal joint.
St 36	Located just lateral to the tibial crest on the lateral aspect of the hind leg.
GB 34	In a depression behind and below the head of the fibula, lateral side of hind leg.
GV 26	Found in the intersection of the 'T' formed below the nose.

131 Key canine acupressure points. (Reproduced by kind permission of Amy Snow, Tallgrass Animal Acupressure Institute, Colorado, USA.)

These techniques have evolved from Swedish massage which, in broad terms, uses long flowing strokes which are divided into several methods of delivery. These are intended to run in parallel with the flow of two of the body's systems: the venous part of the vascular system and the lymphatic system. This has various physiological and psychological effects on the body. Massage works on a cellular basis, and this must be fully understood by the masseur. Moving the hands over the skin, which is highly innervated, has an immediate impact on the connective tissues. These tissues are contiguous throughout the body. Understanding this, and the contraindications to the use of massage, is crucial before any treatment can take place. Skin is the conduit between the therapist and the recipient. Peripheral nerves in the skin carry impulses from sensory receptors such as pressure, pain, temperature, and stretching (see Chapter 2) to the brain, which in turn causes a reaction to occur in an appropriate system or receptive tissue. During massage, these sensory neurons carry stimuli from the skin to the CNS and a response is then transmitted back from the brain to the peripheral nerves and thence to the targeted muscle. In appropriate situations, massage influences cellular exchange that benefits recovery and positive change within the recipient's body. In fact, massage can take over certain cellular responses and render others less active, e.g. during recovery from overexertion, illness, or even maldigestion.

Mechanical techniques

By incorporating mechanical techniques into treatment, the therapist hopes to:

- Enhance venous flow.
- Enhance lymphatic drainage.
- Realign muscle fibres.
- Adjust tissue tension.

These principles have a direct effect on muscle and fascia that may be compromised. By nourishing these cells with the constituents that are required for metabolism, they can then resume normal activity. By providing this to inactive cells, whether caused by damage, physical restriction, or neural restriction, the body can begin its self-healing processes. Throughout this book, the benefits of massage are discussed in relation to influencing venous return and the importance of enhancing the removal of toxins within the venous blood. This encourages arterial blood to flush the area with oxygenated blood that is required for healing. All cells require a stimulus for healthy metabolism. This can be achieved through physical, chemical, or electrical (neural) means; with magnetism; or through other forms of electrotherapy, like ultrasound or low-level laser beams.

Interstitial fluid is a solution which bathes and surrounds the cells of the dog's body, providing another mechanism for nourishing the cells and removing waste; this is done through its interrelationship with the lymphatic system. This system is controlled through osmosis. Many of the surrounding tissues have tiny pores in the cells that this fluid passes through; these can become thick and fibrous with wear and injury. Through mechanical massage, these structures can be kept pliable and maintain good osmotic conditions.

Scar tissue is formed in muscle tissue in a similar way to its formation in skin. However, the scarring in muscle is obviously not visible, and the effects can be both short- and long-term. If the scar tissue is excessive, a chronic inflammatory condition can result, which creates yet more scar tissue. The muscle then becomes calcified, and this can make it feel as hard as bony tissue. The use of more direct manipulative methods, i.e. mechanical massage, plus that of reflexive techniques, can assist the process of breaking down the calcified muscle cells into smaller particles that will be viewed as toxins by the body. They will then be removed by phagocytes within the lymphatic and circulatory systems.

Adhesions and fibrous tissue are another product of injury; again, they can either be acute or chronic (repetitive strain). The healing process of the muscle has several phases during which the tissue can take on a sticky consistency, very similar to a cut hand pre-granulation. During this stage, damaged tissues may adhere to adjoining tissues, especially if mobility within the area is limited. Adhesions can occur in most structures within the body, e.g. muscle to fascia (**132, 133**), muscle to adjacent bone, muscle to adjacent muscle, or muscle to adjacent ligament or tendon.

Within all these situations, the prospect of reduced mobility is high, resulting from reduced range of movement or reduced contractility of one or both structures. Mechanical methods of massage can gently start to break down these adhesions. Rolling and lifting techniques can assist the separation of adhered muscles within groups by physically separating them. This can cause serious pain, and should only be attempted with caution. Passive movement will assist with regaining the proper range of movement.

Fibrous tissue is caused by injury and/or chronic insult to a muscle or muscle group. It can be caused by injury, in which there is a serious muscle fibre tear, or continual damage from repeated untreated microtrauma or overuse. In the case of acute injury, fibres will begin healing, but the new fibres will not resemble the original ones. These fibres will, to varying degrees, lose their contractile quality, because their gliding function will be severely impaired. This gliding function allows the contraction and relaxation of a muscle and, depending on how many fibres have been damaged,

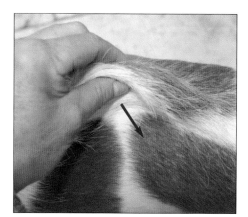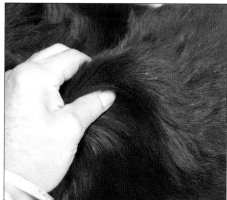

132, 133 The pinch test, used to indicate restricted skin mobilization due to adhesions.

will directly affect the appearance and function of that area. The effect will be the bunching of fibres in an irregular formation that will take on the characteristics of a hard lump or knot. The lack of pliability and flexibility within the area will lead to a restriction of movement and function. During this process, secondary adhesions can also form, thereby adding to the dysfunction of the surrounding tissues.

Transverse stroke and friction can help with this condition; it is worth noting that the process is painful, as by causing friction, the intention is to aggravate the area; therefore, the pain will be great. This is required because compacted and entwined tissue does not have a good circulation. Therefore, to assist with the return of good blood flow and to promote a separation of structures requires a deep mechanical and reflexive technique so that the tissues can begin to regain mobility.

Microtrauma is where small areas of muscle fibre have been damaged. Repair is encouraged by strength training to develop cellular potency through the breaking down (in a measured way) of the damaged fibres and the subsequent remodelling of stronger and more resilient muscle fibres. It can almost be unperceivable to an observer that any trauma has occurred. However, microtrauma is now thought to be the greatest cause of post-event soreness. This trauma, if it is on a small scale, can be fairly innocuous, but if performance dogs are not managed with the correct post-event treatments, these can escalate, causing chronic problems.

Reflexive techniques

Reflexive techniques are ones that are aimed at influencing the nervous and endocrine (hormonal) systems. The nervous system is affected by everything in the dog's environment, so cannot be put in isolation. Likewise, the endocrine system is always trying to achieve homeostasis; therefore, this is constantly feeding back information via the nervous system to achieve these ends.

On a sensory level, the mechano-receptors respond to touch, pressure, warmth, and stretching. These have a reflexive effect which modulates tissue tension and reduces pain. When a body is experiencing pain through tension, the body reacts by promoting an overactive state (survival technique) and the sympathetic nervous system becomes dominant, placing the dog in a constant state of stress. By releasing the tension, the neural response is to stimulate the parasympathetic system; this con-sequently encourages digestive processes and gaseous exchange.

By incorporating reflexive techniques, the parasympathetic and sympathetic nervous systems (sedating or stimulating) are balanced and positively influence neural receptors, including proprioceptors, within the musculoskeletal system. Balancing the parasympathetic and sympathetic nervous systems helps to restore the body to a state between relaxation and excitement. Relaxing the dog through reflexive measures or the relief of underlying pain, allows the autonomic nervous system to function more appropriately. Stimulating the motor neural system or influencing the sympathetic nervous system can help in the preparation for activity (see Chapter 4). By easing pain perception, and by releasing the pressure on nerves or reducing damage to them, we can facilitate the re-establishment of neural pathways that will help to improve tone and spatial awareness. This can lead to huge improvements when the neural activity has been impaired. The release of contorted muscle fibres surrounding nerves can cause a massive improvement in proprioception.

It is also said that by using techniques involving a form of vibration such as tapotment, the pain pathways can be interrupted. This is known as the 'gate control theory' of pain.

The environment and therapist positioning

For a successful treatment, the environment has to be correct. It has to be conducive for a dog to feel both safe and comfortable. Many have not enjoyed their experiences at veterinary surgeries, so it is ideal if the environment does not smell or resemble that of a surgery. If the treatment has to be performed in a veterinary surgery, then it is recommended that changes are made; for example, a large mat could be put on the floor. This may be a fairly subtle change to us, but it can be profound to a dog.

Safety is one of the key objectives when designing an environment. Some therapists prefer to work at a table; however, the dog may not remain perfectly still and could leap or fall off the table. Also, when working with infirm or veteran dogs, putting them on a surface that is not firm causes them to be extremely anxious, and therefore unable to relax. A good compromise is to use a low sofa or something else that will be both comfortable and safe for the dog and practitioner. For those dogs that have the privilege of sleeping on a sofa at home, it helps them to relax, and for those that are not allowed to, it feels like a treat. The other advantage is that if a dog should fall off the surface, the distance is minimal and no injury should be sustained. The floor should be both firm and level so that even the most unstable dog can get a good foothold and stand comfortably. The temperature of the room should be approximately 20°C (65°F), and the size of the room should allow for all sizes of dog to fully extend the thoracic and pelvic limbs.

Self-preservation should always be considered when working in a professional capacity! Although working at a table, as discussed, would be easier for the therapist, due to safety aspects for the dog, working on the floor is more likely. Therefore, it is important that the therapist:

- Ensures that the most appropriate techniques can be applied.
- Avoids taking a dominant stance over the dog.
- Ensures that their position does not incur repetitive strain injuries.
- Breathes properly while treating a dog, so as to help their own muscles to function and not become fatigued.
- Positions themself as comfortably as possible, so that the position is sustainable for anything up to 10 minutes of uninterrupted treatment.

Before beginning to treat a dog, it is important to have the right mindset and that a positive intention is displayed. Showing 'intent' is the equivalent of a polite welcome and introduction to the treatment. Speaking directly to the dog in front of the handler can induce an extremely positive response from a dog, forming a direct connection with it, and showing very deliberate intention and honesty.

Massage application

Pressure

There is no definitive answer as to how much pressure should be applied during treatment, as there is no fixed equation (**134**). It depends on the size of dog and each dog's own tolerance and situation. The golden rule is to start with one pressure, then check for reactions. If the dog is happy and working with the therapist, depending on the conditions, slightly more pressure may be applied. If the dog leans in, that indicates that a little more pressure is required. It is incorrect to think that the greater the pressure, the greater the effect, more often than not, 'less is more'. The therapist should always look to the dog for feedback, as the dog will feedback more than anyone can write on the subject.

Rhythm

A good rhythm is vital when applying a massage; the rhythm and speed are completely dependent on what the objectives are. To sedate the dog for remedial purposes, one stroke per second would be reasonable and the therapist should look to work slightly more slowly than a normal heart rate (70–120 beats per minute) to encourage relaxation. However, to excite the dog, pre-exercise, then a rate of twice that would sensible. Again, watching for signs from the dog will inform whether the rhythm is correct or not.

Number of applications

If effleurage is the technique being used, then the recommended number of repeated applications over one area is three. However, this is not definitive, as there are so many variables that come into the equation, such as:

- How tender is the area?
- Will the dog remain still?
- Is the area one that the dog wants to be worked over?
- Is it an area the dog is keen to guard?

As with many aspects of treatment, the correct answer is decided by the recipient and the therapist's own intuition and experience.

Palpation

'To treat is comparatively easy; it is diagnosis that is difficult'.

Palpation, James Cyriax MD (widely regarded as the father of Orthopaedics).

To learn sensory perception through the hands and its interpretation is one of the most important parts of the education of any practitioner, and one that needs to be developed. Palpation is a real skill and one that can be learnt, but not by everyone. It takes time and practice to develop the skills accurately so that one can assess what is happening beneath the hands. Identifying tissue changes by texture, tension, or irregularity when the surface is covered by a thick layer of hair and skin is not easy. This difficulty is made worse if the recipient is not courteous

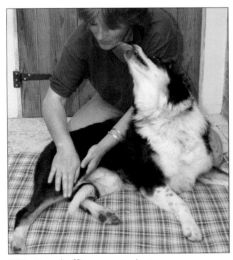

134 Good effleurage technique.

enough to stand, sit, or lie still. At least with a human patient, there can be some verbal feedback, and the request to keep still is usually obeyed! For a new practitioner, learning to read correctly the slight temperature changes that occur with tissue dysfunction takes time and practice; this frustrates many students. Also, a holistic examination must also be part of the process, taking in every slight movement or reaction when the hands pass over each area.

The pressure used must be appropriate; sometimes it is necessary for deeper examination to be performed, and then the overlying tissues must be warmed and prepared. Lameness or tenderness presenting in one area may not necessarily mean that is where the problem lies; it could be the true site of the trauma, or the original insult could be in another area altogether. At other times, the lightest touch can detect what is happening below the surface. Irregularities of texture or temperature can indicate the problem, but there may also be excessive fascial tension within an area. Having the ability to identify this, together with the direction pull requires good tactile skills.

The story below, although fictitious, demonstrates the importance of palpation skills, and how being able to identify where the source of the problem is, is the key to good results.

Once the therapist has developed their palpation skills, the best effects are achieved by those who can 'feel' their way, using their intuition. Once mastered, this is invaluable to a practitioner.

A FAVOURITE STORY

A factory producing millions of high value 'widgets' per hour suddenly came to a crashing halt, resulting in zero production and amounting to massive accumulative losses. The machinery failed to work and the factory's maintenance man could not find the problem. The factory owner stated that if anyone could find someone who could repair the machinery he would pay that repair man £100,000.

One employee made a call to a friend who duly arrived at the factory with just a small tool-carrying belt and demanded a ladder to ascend the offending inoperative machine. When he reached the top, he stopped, looked, listened, moved very slightly, and hit the machine a hefty blow with his hammer. The machinery churned into action and resumed producing the 'widgets'. He descended the ladder and made his way to the factory owner's office.

'Here is a bill for £100,000 to repair your machine', said the repair man.

'What!' said the factory owner, 'I am not paying you £100,000 just to simply hit my machine with a hammer!'

'Ok,' said the repair man, 'here are two bills: one for £10 for hitting your machine with my hammer, and one for £99,990 for knowing where to hit it!'

Anon

Massage techniques

The divisions within massage technique are explained differently in practically every textbook on massage; this is why it is not necessarily important to remember the names, but it is essential to know what they do and what the effects are. Techniques include:

- Effleurage.
- Petrissage.
- Friction.
- Tendon release.
- Tapotment.
- Passive movement.
- Passive touch.

Please note: massage should not be attempted without practical tuition.

Effleurage

The word 'effleurage' derives from a French word, effeurer, meaning 'to touch lightly'. It is a gentle sweeping stroke made with the flat of the hand. Within a Swedish massage routine, it is the technique used to open and close; in other words, to begin and end a treatment. For this, the hands must contour over the underlying tissue, and sweeping movements are used that are slow and rhythmic, with a confident touch that can be applied by one or two hands.

The pressure being exerted (**135**) must be even over the whole of the hand's surface, with the fingers remaining together and the thumb following the direction of the fingers. The strokes generally run the full length of the muscles with a speed to enable recognition of tissue texture and tension. For smaller dogs, two or three fingers can be used instead of the whole hand (**136**). Equal pressure should be used, without more asserted through the fingertips. Slightly more pressure can be applied after the initial routine has been established. The uses and advantages of this technique are many; not least, it forms the initial contact between therapist and dog, and is key to the formation of a positive relationship and trust between the two. It is also used as a joining technique, and can be used in many situations.

One of the main intentions when performing effleurage is to influence venous and lymphatic return. It has a mechanical effect of assisting their

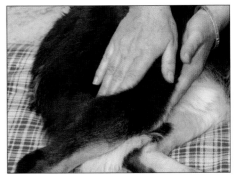

135 Effleurage.

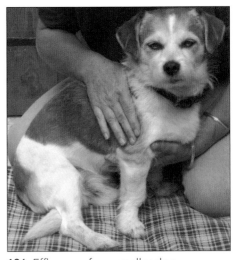

136 Effleurage for a smaller dog.

movement, by apparently replicating muscle movement, and also targeting problem areas. By influencing venous drainage, arterial flow in the area is enhanced, bringing an increase in the amounts of oxygen and nutrition that are brought to the area; this will also enhancing warming of the area. The influence on the lymphatic system can aid lymphatic drainage and return (see Chapter 2). The speed or rhythm of the stroke can also have an effect of relaxation or calming, if applied slowly, or a more invigorating effect, if applied faster.

It is possibly one of the most versatile of all the techniques as many aspects of the basic technique can be varied, including pressure (superficial or deep) and direction of application, according to the muscle fibre direction (longitudinal or transverse). Superficial effleurage is used for the introductory strokes, and works on a superficial level, using light pressure. Deep effleurage follows superficial or light effleurage, when the pressure is adjusted to work more deeply, to influence the deeper tissues. It does not mean more force is applied, just a smaller working area may be used. Longitudinal application, together with superficial pressure, is the technique most treatments begin with. This can be repeated over an area several times. In transverse application, the strokes are applied across the direction of the muscle fibres. This is a good diagnostic method, as at times fibrous tissue can run with the line of the muscle fibre, and it is not until it is crossed that the area can be identified.

Key points for application of effleurage

- The technique applications include: one-handed, hand-over-hand.
- It can be applied superficially or deeply.
- It can be applied longitudinally or transversely.
- It is used as an opening technique at the start of a massage or throughout the massage in conjunction with additional massage techniques.
- It can influence the movement of blood in the dog's body and promote venous and lymphatic return and cellular interchange.
- It can be applied to the cheeks, ears, top and sides of the head, trunk, back and pelvic region, thoracic and pelvic limbs.
- It is applied with the palms of the hands, fingers, or fingertips (depending on the size of the dog).
- The hand, fingers, or fingertips should slide readily and evenly over the dog's coat.
- Even pressure should be maintained for the entire stroke and from one stroke to the next; the pressure can slightly increase as muscles warm and if the recipient is happy.
- It is an excellent assessment tool for identifying change/s in tissue before and after superficial tissues have been warmed.

Petrissage

'Petrissage' comes from the French word, pétrir, meaning to knead or rub. This stroke forms a name for a collective group of techniques, and has the overall objective of manipulating tissues by rubbing and kneading, using the pressure of the hands or fingers to break down any tension. This technique is only used when the tissues have been warmed, and not on bony or delicate areas.

The rationale for this group of techniques is to produce a local compression followed by a release that can influence both the superficial and deep tissues on the dog's body. By constricting blood flow to the local area, then releasing it, the body reacts by flooding the area with fresh arterial blood. The pressure employed when applying this technique should begin very lightly and can then be increased as the tissue warms and the patient becomes accustomed to the procedure.

The primary objective of superficial petrissage is to stimulate all functions of the skin, e.g. to influence venous return and to empty and refill the lymph spaces beneath the skin. Deep petrissage has a good effect on releasing superficial fascial adhesions; this, however, must be done using care, as it can be extremely painful. Superficial kneading is applied to the coat so as to influence the skin. It can be applied in a random pattern all over the coat, or upwards or downwards.

Superficial kneading
Skin rolling
This superficial technique can be extremely relaxing for a dog; however, caution should be used if it is used over areas of fascial tension, as the area will be tender. It can be applied anywhere, but mainly over the cranial and dorsal regions where the skin should be loose and can be grasped easily (**137, 138**); other good target areas include sites of old wounds. However, care must be taken not to pinch the skin and, if the skin is tight or sticky, not to lift too much, as this feels the same as pulling a sticking plaster off exposed flesh.

In this technique:

- The skin is grasped gently between thumb and the flat of the fingers.
- The fingers are moved forward in small incremental steps – as if they are 'walking', followed by the thumb 'walked' up behind the fingers.
- The skin will respond in a wave-like motion.
- With tight skin, the technique should be performed slowly and sympathetically.

If this is done over loose skin (**137**), it is a relaxing and enjoyable treatment. However, if the skin is tight and adhered to the tissue below (**138**), it will be painful; care must be taken in choosing where and when the technique is applied.

Plucking
If applied correctly, this can be extremely relaxing and useful as a calming technique:

- A few hairs of the coat nearest to the hair follicle are grasped between one or two fingers and the thumb.
- The fingers are slid up the shaft of the hair fairly quickly (not pulling the hair); the hair is then released the top of the hair is reached.
- Alternate hands are used to work an entire area of the dog, grasping, sliding, and releasing, to simulate a plucking motion.

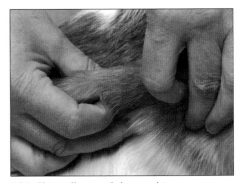

137 Skin rolling with loose skin.

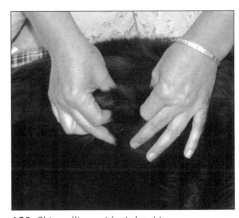

138 Skin rolling with tight skin.

- Care should be taken not to pinch or pull the hair too rigorously.
- Plucking should be applied slowly at first, then increased to a fairly quick rate, adjusted to each individual dog's comfort level.

Deep kneading

The primary objective is to bring blood and nutrients to the belly of the muscle, to release toxins, and to relax muscle spasms trapped within a specific muscle or group of muscles. It can also be used for muscle fibre realignment, affecting muscle length and congruity. It is applied with the hands, fingers, or finger tips, relatively quickly and lightly to cover the entire muscle.

Friction

Like many anatomical words, this derives from a Latin word, fricare, which means to rub or to rub down (**139**), and sometimes is classed as petrissage. Friction is a variation of rubbing, and work by locally compressing tissue against bone, using a single fingertip to irritate the underlying tissues by using short cross-fibre movements. This, too, should never be used before all the surrounding tissues have been thoroughly warmed. Friction is an excellent technique for working around bony protrusions, e.g. either side of the vertebrae, the head, face, and any irregular shape:

- The fingertips are placed on the tissue and moved in a circular constant motion, while lightly pressing inwards.
- The fingers are held close together to maintain control while the thumb is used as a stabilizing point.
- To go deeper into the fibres, a slower rate is used but not heavier pressure; a light touch is maintained throughout; then the pressure is released.
- This technique can be applied transversely, longitudinally, or circularly.

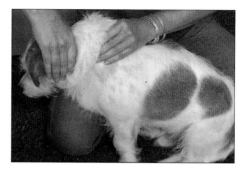

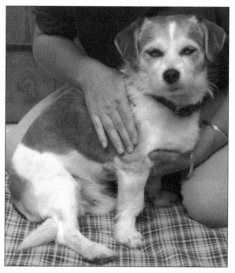

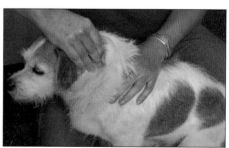

139 Digital kneading (friction).

Friction should be applied extremely sympathetically, as the areas that will require a frictional technique will be the most tender and sensitive. The idea of friction is to cause an irritation by causing a minor inflammatory effect; therefore, it is an acute response. By provoking this reaction, the area will become mildly erythemic, causing an increase of heat within the area. Frictional techniques are intended also to break down contorted muscle fibre that surrounds nerves. The nerves will be restricted or heightened in perception, so care should be taken at all times. Important: this technique should only be applied for a few seconds at a time.

Compression

Compression (**140**) is good for the larger muscles or muscle groups; the therapist:

- Locates the belly of the muscle and places the palm of the hand, fingers, or fingertips on the belly of the muscle.
- The muscle is gently pressed in a rhythmic pumping action, holding the compression for approximately 1–2 seconds.
- Additional pressure is applied progressively as the tissues warm and soften; the dog's reaction should be monitored during this time.
- When one area becomes warm and softens, another area is worked on, or another technique is used.
- The limb being worked on should always be supported.

Picking up

Picking up (**141**) can be applied to any muscle or muscle groups that can be grasped, lifted, or rolled. This is generally mostly appreciated by the dog when it is used over the neck, shoulder, and over the loose skin of the back. The therapist:

- Grasps the muscle, compressing the tissue lightly between the thumb and the flat of the fingers.

- Gently lifts the tissue, slightly rolling the hand away from the body, and releases it.
- Alternate hand are used to build up a rhythm.

Finger stripping or thumb glide

Finger stripping or thumb glide (**142, 143**) can be performed longitudinally following the length of long muscles and alongside the vertebrae of the dog. The therapist:

- Places the fingers or the pad of the thumb on the muscle.
- Gently presses inward and glides along the entire length of the muscle in the direction of the muscle fibres.
- Continues the passes until all the fibres have been covered, starting lightly and increasing the pressure.

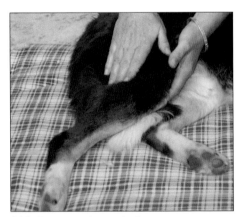

140 Compression technique.

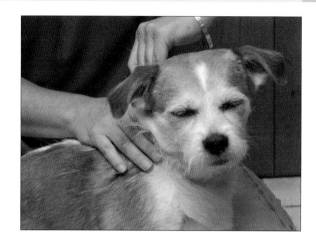

141 Picking up is especially welcome over the neck and scapula regions.

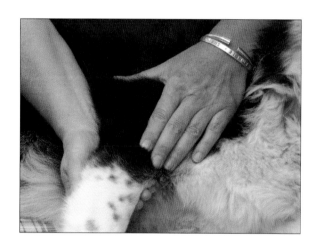

142 Thumb glide, working longitudinally down the m. triceps brachii.

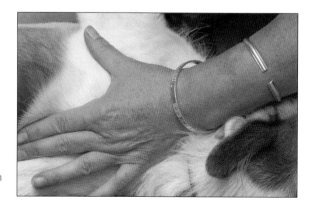

143 Finger glide, working down the paravertebral muscles.

Cross-fibre working

Cross-fibre working (**144–146**) is exactly as its name implies, so this must be used with care over any possible sites of chronic injury. It should only be applied to the large articulating muscles. A variety of techniques can be used in this method:

- Single-handed:

  - The back of the fingers are placed on the dog so that the fingers line up with the direction of the muscle fibres.
  - The muscles are compressed and then the hand is rotated up to a 90° position.
  - The knuckles will be moving in an outward direction, the right thumb will travel in a clockwise direction.
  - For smaller dogs or muscles, the same technique as above is used but with just two fingers rotating (**144**).
  - For single-handed fibre spread the palm of the hand is placed against the dog's muscles with the fingers aligned with the muscle fibres, and the technique is executed by rotation of the base of the hand in an outward direction against the line of the fibres.
  - Two-handed fibre spread (**145, 146**)
  - Using the flat tips of the fingers or thumbs, the hands are moved in opposite directions (apart) across the muscle fibre.

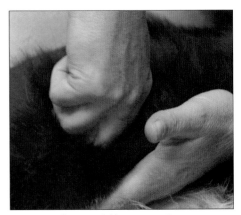

144 Two-fingered fibre spread.

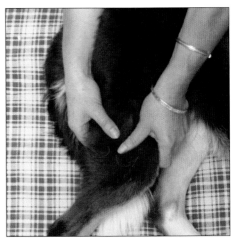

145 Fibre spread on a larger dog.

Tendon release

Tendon release (**147, 148**) is a technique which is beneficial for muscles and tendons of the thoracic and pelvic limbs. The technique uses one hand while the other supports the limb in an extended position. The working hand grasps the fleshy portion of the muscle and works along the axis of the limb with short up and down motions. The movement should

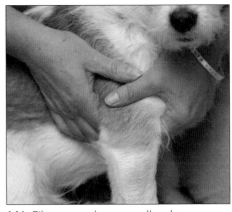

146 Fibre spread on a smaller dog.

be continuous and smooth, being careful not to pinch the muscle or skin.

Tapotment

Tapotment covers a number of techniques which consist of a light vibration, e.g. hacking and cupping, to produce stimulatory signals to the tissues of the body. This is perhaps the technique that is used least; however, it is highly effective in the correct situation. Hacking is applied by the outside surface of the little finger of one or both hands, striking the muscle in a random pattern, with loose relaxed wrist. If the technique is being conducted correctly, a very slight 'slapping' of fingers will be heard. Cupping is also applied with loose wrists and hands, forming a 'cup', which is intended to trap air between the hand and the dog's body. This is again applied in a random pattern and, if applied correctly, a hollow clapping sound will be heard.

Please note: all of these tapotment techniques should only be applied over dense muscle or muscle groups, and only after instruction; incorrectly used tapotment can feel like a slap or a punch.

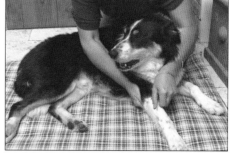

147 Tendon release technique.

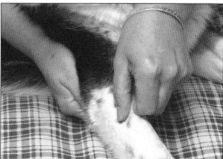

148 Photo showing the gentle ease and release required in tendon release.

Passive movements

This is the movement of an articulating joint without active participation by the dog. The use of passive movement within a massage routine is extremely important both for the active and less active dog; it can be both part of the assessment and of the treatment (see Chapter 4). The aim is to take the target joint through its natural anatomical range, or to the 'end feel'. If the joint is compromised in some way, the same applies: the joint must only go through its possible range, not the potential range. The joint works in close collaboration with the adjoining soft tissues that facilitate its stable and smooth articulation.

For full range of function, the following structures are necessary:

- Cartilaginous surfaces: should be smooth and concussion-receiving surfaces.
- The synovial fluid: should provide lubrication of the moving structures.
- The external and internal ligaments that restrain and contain the joint.
- Muscles that provide the force to allow the joints to become levers.

This programme stimulates the neural pathways of the joint as a whole. It actively promotes increased movement and flexibility, by influencing the Golgi tendon receptors within the tendons and the muscle spindles within the muscles, plus all the stretch reflex receptors within the ligaments. It is also believed that replicating movement of the joint assists the formation of synovial fluid, which can help prevent:

- Cartilage erosion, through the loss of lubricants (proteoglycans) and a change of structure.
- The release of free radicals, leading to further change and damage.

- Cartilage changes; it changes from being a stiff gel, and becomes more brittle as it loses water.
- An increase in the amount of friction between bones, leading to the destruction of articular cartilage.

If passive movement is performed correctly, it will also help with neural reprogramming of all the soft tissue adjacent to the joint. To execute this safely without causing problems, all the articulating joints must be carefully supported before and during the movements being made. It can also be incorporated into warm-up and warm-down routines, but there are some very strict rules that have to be adhered to. In remedial cases, it is advisable to perform with the dog lying supine, but in any case, the dog must be fully supported and secure.

When using this technique:

- It is crucial that the joints and tissues have been sufficiently warmed by effleurage.
- The dog must be comfortable and stable, either standing or lying.
- Passive movement involves taking the joint through its natural anatomical movement. It is not a stretch.
- The passive movement should be conducted slowly so that all the tissues involved have time to adjust without any sudden or erratic movement. If a joint is moved quickly, damage to the muscle and joint can be inflicted.
- The joint should be held in position (flexed or extended) for at least 15–20 seconds.
- After every movement, the joint is taken back to a neutral point and held there before the next passive movement is applied.
- No more than three passive moves for each joint should be performed.

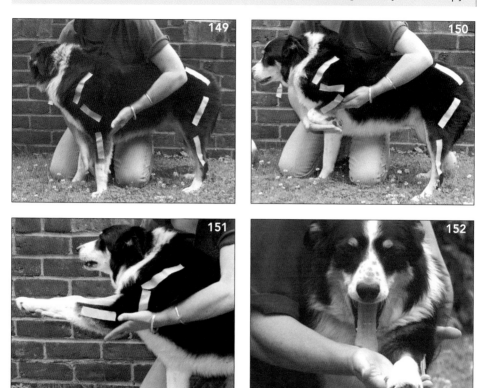

149–152 Passive movement of the thoracic limb. Tape showing angulation of the scapulohumeral and elbow joints (149), showing the change in these angles. 150: Flexion of the scapulohumeral, elbow, and carpal joints: the flexion is achieved by easing the elbow dorsally and medially. The carpus is gently flexed; 151, 152: protraction of the shoulder and extension of thoracic limb showing the increased angle of the scapulohumeral joint, and extension of front leg at carpus.

- All the moving limbs must be supported above and below the joints.
- Passive movement must not be used by an open wound, on a freshly injured site, by any swelling, or to a locked joint.
- After passive movement, effleurage/light exercise is used to readjust joints and tissues.

Please note: this can be used on arthritic joints, but only to the range of movement of that particular joint. Passive movements of the thoracic limb are shown in Figures 149–152. Note that the elbow is the joint where the leg is eased forwards from, not pulled from the carpus. Note that the leg is drawn directly in front of the dog, neither adducting nor abducting.

Passive movements of the pelvic limb are shown in Figures **153–156**. The stifle is gently extended (in a large dog, the hock must be supported), not pulling through the hock. The hand must support the stifle in all dogs, and the limb is extended in a direct line with the dog's body.

Passive touch

This is a valuable technique for the nervous dog or one in pain. It can be used as an opening technique as it introduces the dog to touch. It has a calming and warming effect as tension is released, that initiates a trust-building environment. It is done with no pressure or movement, just a gentle touch using the palm of the hands or fingers placed lightly on the body. Some dogs who are extremely resistant to touch find it less intrusive if the back of the hand is used. It can be used anywhere on the body, and hands or fingertips are left in place for about 30–90 seconds (*Table 15*).

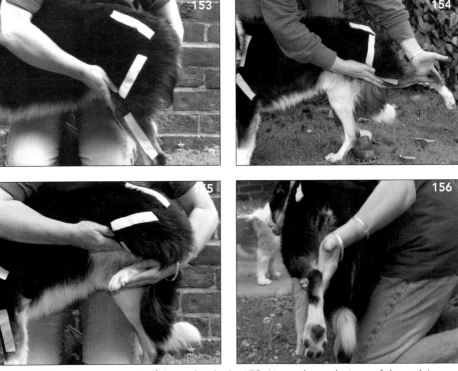

153–156 Passive movement of the pelvic limb. **153**: Normal angulations of the pelvis, femur, and tibia. **154**: flexion of the stifle and pelvis. Note how the stifle and hock are protected and the femoral pelvic joint eased into a flexed position through gentle pressure through the stifle. **155, 156**: extension of the stifle and pelvis, executed by easing the stifle through the extension.

Table 15 Summary of massage techniques, purposes, and effects

Technique	Purpose	Mechanical effect	Reflexive effect
Superficial effleurage (superficial stroking) • A smooth gliding action using the whole hand to cover a large surface area • Two hands may be used, or alternate hands in a slow rhythmic motion • Working on the superficial muscle layer with the hand/s following fibre direction of the underlying muscle • The pressure should be light initially, gradually increasing as the underlying tissues warm	• To adjust the dog to touch and to demonstrate 'intent' • Used at the start of a treatment: • To warm the area • To relax the muscles • To assist drainage of the venous blood • To assist drainage of the lymphatic system • To evaluate current and changing state of tissue • Can also be used as a transitioning stroke between other techniques to maintain relaxation, particularly following deep tissue massage	• Warms the tissue and muscle fibres through frictional warmth, influencing venous return, then promoting arterial interchange • Stimulates the lymphatic system by replicating gentle muscle movement • Gently eases myofascial connections	Works on the parasympathetic nervous system and relaxes muscles • Venous and arterial capillary circulation is enhanced • Endorphins are released, giving pain relief; this also aids relaxation • Soothes nerve endings within the skin
Deep effleurage (deep stroking) • As above but following light effleurage working slightly more deeply with slightly more pressure, both transversely or longitudinally to the muscle fibre direction	• Used to work deeper into the tissue and muscle fibres on specific, localized areas of tension or injury sites • Can be used as a stretching mechanism for the muscle fibres	• Warms superficial tissue, enhances vasodilatation and causing mild erythema • Warms tissues to allow for 'deeper' techniques mild erythema	

(continues)

Table 15 Summary of massage techniques, purposes, and effects (continued)

Technique	Purpose	Mechanical effect	Reflexive effect
Deep effleurage (deep stroking) • Smaller surfaces of the hand are used (or larger areas with greater pressure) in order to concentrate the pressure, using thumb pad; finger pads; ulna surface of the fist; palm heel • The tendons and attachment points should be included as well as the belly of the muscle, with strokes directed towards the belly of the muscle in order to stretch the tendon; this also induces muscle relaxation • Transverse stroking is used primarily as a diagnostic technique to identify localized muscle tension; it is conducted across the belly of the muscle using the flat area of the hands or fingers	• Assessment tool for palpation of deeper tissues	• Assists further the removal of metabolic waste and can reduce oedema by influencing venous and lymphatic return and assisting the flow of arterial blood • Assists cellular exchange and thus health • Assists the nutritional status of the tissues • Sheds the outer layers of dead skin, and can stimulate sebum production • Realigns muscle fibres to promote correct healing/placement	• Promotes homeostasis by creating a more relaxed dog, influencing the parasympathetic nervous system • Can be used to promote excitement by influencing the sympathetic nervous system

Table 15 Summary of massage techniques, purposes, and effects (continued)

Technique	Purpose	Mechanical effect	Reflexive effect
Petrissage (deep kneading) • Both hands are used to apply kneading in a rhythmical way • Using alternate hands the muscle or muscle group is lifted away from the underlying structure	• Often used after effleurage: • To relieve congestion • To reduce swelling • To help prevent muscle shortening through excessive use	• Stretches and realigns muscle fibres, stimulates muscle tone • Breaks down adhesions • Circulation and elimination of waste is enhanced • Drainage of excess interstitial fluid is assisted	• Relaxes the nervous system with slow movement • Stimulates the nervous system with fast movement • Affects proprioceptive sense through release of neural pathways

Picking up:
- Hands gently encircle an area (typically the neck) and in a rhythmic wave action the fingers are drawn up and lifted through the muscle tissue, alternating the hand at the top and the hand at the bottom of the area.
- To relieve muscle fibre congestion
- To ease tension through shortening of muscle fibres
- To ease tension of overload muscle fibres
- To assist the separation of congested fibres
- To apply a direct stretch over the muscle tissue
- To help break down scar tissue
- Relaxing effect through easing of pain perception

(continues)

Table 15 Summary of massage techniques, purposes, and effects (continued)

Technique	Purpose	Mechanical effect	Reflexive effect
Friction • The pads of the thumbs or fingertips are used • Application is only on localized problem areas once the tissues have been warmed up • There are different techniques used in applying friction massage: • Circular, applied using the thumb or individual fingers in a transverse or circular motion to give a slow frictional movement	• Used to break down scar tissue or treat hard muscle bands that have resulted from overuse or injury • Treatment of hypertonic muscle spasm • Remedial treatment of acute injuries • Deep tissue work; often used around the joints to break down fibrosis and stimulate circulation • Also used to break down inflexible scar tissue	• Separates adhered fascial planes (myofascial release) • Realigns muscle fibres • Breaks down adhesions • Helps break down scar tissue and promotes the formation of more tolerable elastic fibrous tissue	• Stimulates appropriate Golgi tendon reflex activity by reducing tension in opposing muscles • Increase circulation and blood flow
Cross-fibre	• To re-align muscle fibres and break down scar and fibrous tissue	• Aids the separation of muscle fibres and fibrous tissue	• Influences positively the muscle spindle stretch receptors within the muscle

Table 15 Summary of massage techniques, purposes, and effects (continued)

Technique	Purpose	Mechanical effect	Reflexive effect
Finger/thumb glide	• To realign muscle fibres, aid vasodilatation, and promote elasticity within the fibres	• Realigns superficial and deep fibres	• Positively influences the muscle spindles, assisting a resumption of appropriate muscle contraction and relaxation
Compression	• To encourage venous exchange gently	• Compression of the fibres within the belly of the muscle, facilitating a mild venous drainage and promoting the flow of arterial blood to the area	• Has a mild relaxation effect and aids homeostasis
Plucking superficial	• To relax the dog and superficial tissues	• Gently manipulates the hair follicles • Causes mild vasodilatation	• Stimulates the parasympathetic nervous system
Skin rolling superficial	• To ease superficial adhesions • Can be used when other mechanical techniques are too uncomfortable • To ease fascial connections	• To ease superficial adhesions • Can be used when other mechanical techniques are too uncomfortable • To ease fascial connections	• Stimulates the parasympathetic nervous system • Helps tighten myofascial bands

(continues)

Table 15 Summary of massage techniques, purposes, and effects (continued)

Technique	Purpose	Mechanical effect	Reflexive effect
Tapotment (percussion) • A rhythmical technique using both hands in a rapid action: • Hacking (with the ulnar surface of the hand) • Cupping (using the hands in a cup-type hold, enabling the trapping of air) • Wrists must always be kept loose	• To stimulate muscles • To relax hypertonic muscles • Helps to promote good muscle tone	• Will influence vasodilatation	• Will excite the sympathetic nervous system
Tendon release	• To maintain carpal flexibility	• Eases the retinaculum of the carpus to facilitate smooth tendon movement • Eases extensor tendons	
Passive movement	• To maintain or enhance range of movement	• Eases joints through their natural range	• Influences the Golgi tendon receptors • Influences the muscle spindles • Enhances the activity of subchondral cell production to improve viscosity of synovial fluid

Assessment of the dog

Introduction
'A strong, even gait is desirable in all breeds no matter the size, the shape, or purpose'.
Rachel Page Elliott

When a healthy, balanced dog moves, it flows. The movements are seamless, connected, and pleasurable to watch. The muscles are moving in phase appropriately, which means that the dog efficiently uses its natural balance, and moves in a sustainable and rhythmic manner.

Dogs are in a multitude of different shapes and sizes, which produce a diverse range of gait patterns. Even though the gait sequence is the same, the footfall will differ, e.g. a trot of a short-legged or achondroplastic dog is not capable of 'tracking up', in comparison to that of a larger, longer-legged dog. There are many variables that affect gait and, more importantly, balance; the art is to determine what can be treated to aid movement, and that which is inherent.

Along with the many variables the therapist needs to consider, certain shoulder and stifle angulations are desirable in certain breeds, as well as length of back and the shape of the top line. As a practitioner, the question: does this shape serve the dog well? should be considered first and foremost, the therapist should be looking for congruence and where the point of incongruence lies.

An overt lameness is easy to assess; one can clearly say 'the dog is lame' if, for example, it was between 5/10 and 10/10 lame. However, the difficultly comes when the dog is 'unsound' but not overtly lame, lacking flow and natural balance, and is anything from 1/10 to 5/10 lame. This may only present in walk, trot, or canter, and may even only occur when the dog rises from rest or at the beginning or the end of exercise. The unsound dog is the one that can be overlooked or, at worst, discounted. This is the dog that is harbouring problems for the future, problems that will start to accumulate through a process of somatic change, and which the dog will ultimately start compensating for, however small the initial problem. These changes will develop exponentially, and are not sustainable in the long term.

Evaluating a dog
When a dog is brought to a practitioner for treatment, it must have had a full physical examination by a veterinary surgeon. In many cases, this examination will have given a clear diagnosis of the problem or a good steer towards something that involves the soft tissues, either primarily or secondarily, and an indication of the possible cause. At any time, when a practitioner is not happy with the dog's response to the treatment, the dog should always be referred back to the veterinary surgeon. In all cases of lameness, whether the dog is overtly lame, intermittently lame, or just unsound, there are many different possible causes, and this is where careful holistic evaluation is so important.

It is all very well having a 'hit list' of areas to evaluate, but what do they mean, and how will they help in the assessment and, therefore, treatment of any client? In all assessments, the external factors presenting and how they relate to breed/type, conformation, lifestyle, and environment must be taken into consideration. Visual evaluation a dog prior to treatment could include:

- Apparent lameness.
- Breed/type.
- Age.
- Overall condition of the dog.
- Balance and footfall.
- Shape of the dog.
- Weightbearing.
- The 'look in the eye'.

Apparent lameness

If the dog displays an apparent lameness, this may not be where the origin lies. The therapist is constantly analysing cause and effect; in other words, is the lameness the main or only problem, is it due to referred pain, or is it a compensatory factor from a problem in another area? Lameness is a good starting point, but it is important to follow through with the rest of the evaluation so as to gain as full a picture as possible before starting any type of treatment. For example, very often an intermittent lameness in the thoracic limbs has origins in the pelvic region.

Breed/type

Breed/type is not going to give any direct indications as to the cause of a problem, but information on the dog's activities and its breed or type, may give a clue; for example, if a miniature Dachshund is presented, the fact that it has been doing agility may suggest possible causes. This is not to say that a Dachshund should not compete in agility, but merely to suggest that its build is more suited to digging and hunting than jumping. This example is extreme and seems obvious, but sometimes the obvious is missed; all the factors that impact on any dog should be considered prior to treatment.

Alternatively, breed stereotyping should also be avoided, in that every Labrador seen with a pelvic limb stiffness does not necessarily have hip dysplasia (without any supporting radiographic evidence), or every German Shepherd dog with compromised proprioception within the same region does not have chronic degenerative radiculomyelopathy (CDRM). These are indicators, but they should not lead a practitioner solely in that particular direction.

Age

Age is sometimes, but not always, relevant; again, it is necessary to go back to the veterinary diagnosis. If a 6–9-month-old giant- or large-breed puppy with thoracic limb lameness is presented, there is a strong possibility that this is a joint issue; therefore, if the dog does not respond very quickly, it should be swiftly referred back to the veterinary surgeon. Usually, age is not a particularly important factor, but the majority of chronic or intermittent cases do seem to fall into the 6–8-year-old age bracket. This is more than likely to be the result of referred pain from a series of microtraumas that has had a slowly progressive detrimental effect. This is a classic problem in the middle-aged dog, and is one that affects both the working dog and the companion dog. A classical case is that of the companion dog that has had a life of minimal weekday exercise, then 4-hour marathons at the weekends. This scenario is one that is not conducive to good muscular condition and health.

If a dog has had a fit and relatively healthy life, it will respond exceptionally well to treatment, even if it is 12+ years old. Sometimes, this category of dog is almost discounted for treatment, because they are old or arthritic and, therefore, it is assumed nothing can help. This may be so, but pain from muscular problems could be a primary or secondary cause of any joint problem, and easing this joint pain will support the primary condition, and also alleviate the stress involved, both physiological and psychological.

Overall condition of the dog

This is a broad statement, but it goes back to the congruence question. Is the dog overweight? What is the coat telling us? Obviously, if the dog is overweight, the possibility of mobility-related issues is increased. Regarding the coat, it is a reflection of what is occurring beneath the surface. A classical example is the dog that presents with a healthy coat, but over a particular area there is some dullness or inconsistency. This abnormal area is a helpful pointer as to where the problem may lie, or, at least, where the stress point may be.

Balance and footfall

How the dog moves through the gaits should be assessed, observing from the side the dog moving away and towards the therapist, and moving on the circle. The whole dog should be observed; are there any areas that lack smoothness, or show an unusual gait pattern? Is there any lateral or medial deviation, or circumduction of the limbs? The stride length should be even and, at a trot, most dogs should 'track up'; in other words, the back foot should land exactly where the front foot was, on both sides. This, obviously, does not occur with achondroplastic dogs, such as Dachshunds and Basset hounds. Look for any weaknesses in the joints; some stifle problems will cause a medial deviation of the joint. A common fault in the show ring is 'weak stifles'; this is a weakness that generally displays no lameness, but can indicate a lack of pelvic and lumbar support. The therapist should watch for any stiffness that is affecting the movement. Lower lumbar stiffness can make the dog look as if it is wearing a filled nappy/diaper; in other words, the legs do not look comfortable in any way. Observe the hip joints; a stiffness in the hip flexors can make a pelvic limb look as if it is being cranked, and not gliding.

The lumbar region is the bridge that joins the back end to the front end. This is a vulnerable part of any animal with a similar skeletal structure to that of the dog. The lumbar region, like any bridge, will reflect imbalances in its supporting structures along its entire length. In Figure 157, the cables represent the myofascial system and the main hard structure of the bridge represents the skeletal system. If any one of the suspension cables is tightened, it will contort the main structure.

In a dog, this region is intended to facilitate the extraordinary ventro-cranial flexion that produces the uplift for a jump and the projection forwards; in a Greyhound, Whippet, and similar breeds, this is particularly exaggerated. If the lumbar region is compromised, it will look stiff and produce a restrained gait. The height of the head is important: does it drop when it engages in movement? This could indicate a neck problem. A nodding action can also denote lameness, as a dog will lift its head when an injured or painful thoracic limb strikes the ground, in an attempt to keep weight off the limb, and it will dip when a lame hindleg strikes the ground. The tail is also worth observing, for as part of the vertebral system it can indicate issues of imbalance or discomfort within the pelvic region, or a lack of overall balance. It can deviate to the left or right, hang like an inverted 'L', or be clasped to the hindlegs. All of these indicate inbalance or a problem within the croup or the lower back.

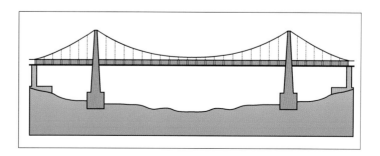

157 A suspension bridge.

Shape of the dog

With all the breeds and crossbreeds, the size and shape of dogs seem to be almost infinitely variable. However, for ease, there seem to be some distinctive body types that can be described:

- The torpedo (**158**, **159**).
- The half-moon (kyphosis or roached back) (**160**).
- The banana (**161**).
- The pelvic slide (dorsal/posterior pelvic tilt) (**162**).
- The misfit (**163**).

These groups are only intended as a guide to assist the training of the eye to look for characteristics that will help detect the source of the problem. These formulated shapes can, in some cases, be further divided into chronic, acute, and subacute:

- Chronic: the chronic cases of shape changes are those in which the muscle patterning has been so disturbed that the dog has developed a unique way of moving and may or may not display an overt lameness.

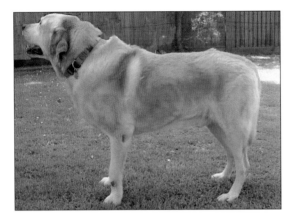 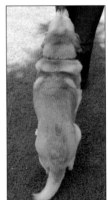

158, 159 Torpedo body shape. **158**: lateral view; **159**: dorsal view.

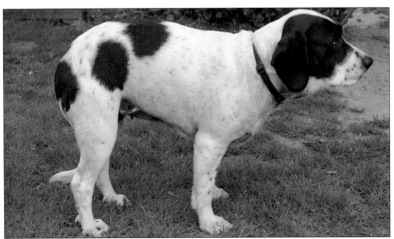

160 Half-moon body shape.

- Acute: in the acute case, the dog is protecting a current injury or persistent pain/discomfort.
- Subacute: this is a situation where an untreated injury is being irritated by an activity and is, thus, causing pain. This may be when jumping or performing some other dynamic action, getting up in the morning or after a period of rest, before or after exercise, or for no apparent reason.

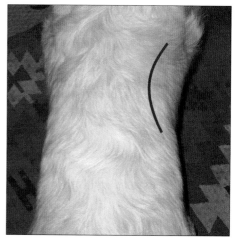

161 Dorsal view of a dog with a mildly banana-shaped back. The line indicates shortened muscles.

162 Pelvic slide with reduced pelvic muscles (arrow).

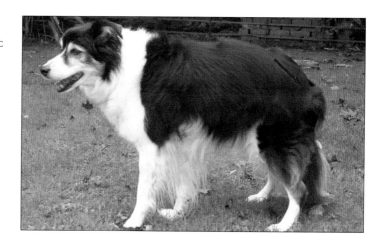

163 The misfit (more apparent through movement).

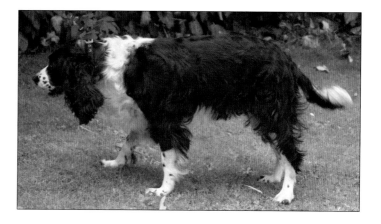

Torpedo shape

This is one of the classic chronic shapes and can be observed from the lateral (**158**) and dorsal (**159**) aspects. The neck and shoulders are thickened, and the pelvic region is tapered, a classic case of total incongruence. These changes have slowly developed because the dog has been finding that propulsion from the front end is less uncomfortable than from the pelvic region, the designated engine, and, therefore, it has adopted 'front wheel drive'. This shape is like a ticking bomb. It is only a matter of time before the overworked thoracic region, mainly intended for the absorption of concussion and directional control, breaks down under the load of supporting 60% of the body weight as well as having the unaccustomed responsibility for mobility.

Half moon

Figure **160** shows a dog with a roached back and slack abdominal muscles, making it look like a half moon. The shape can be less marked than this. It is demonstrated both at the stand and during movement. This shape can be chronic, subacute, or acute. It is generally caused by a deep lumbar problem that gives the impression that the dog has a roached back. This is not to be confused with the natural shape of the Greyhound, Whippet, or Italian Greyhound and other such breeds, that are built with a rather pronounced curvature of the lumbar region to facilitate enhanced propulsion. In these breeds, the normal dog appears almost to have a roached back. This shape displays obvious pelvic and lumbar stiffness and will also produce premature fatiguing (as with most of these shapes), owing to the muscles working inappropriately. Obvious heat is often felt emanating from the T10–12 area, as this is the typical stress point. It is also often connected with a dog 'pacing'. This is a gait where the two right legs protract and then retract together, followed by the two left legs, splitting the pace into two equal halves down the midline rather than on the diagonal. It is easier for a dog with a roached back to employ a pace which produces less stress across the diagonal, so the dog can adopt a rolling action to aid propulsion, rather than having direct drive from the back end. As previously mentioned, dogs with this body type fall into three categories:

- Chronic; this can be viewed as the 'monster lying beneath', being just as insidious as the subacute. One must wonder how long the stress on the T10–13 region can be sustained. Is it a coincidence that many dogs with either induced or inherent thoraco-lumbar disc disease present with similar symptoms? It is well documented that disc disease most commonly occurs in this region, the onset being gradual or acute with the dog showing reluctance to run, jump, or climb stairs.

- Acute: this could be displayed as a guarding device against a lower lumbar pain, from a dynamic injury, from a fall, or even post-operatively. Some dogs which are cryptorchid and then castrated (leaving one retained intra-abdominal testicle) will portray this shape post-operatively, possibly due to deep lumbar muscular disturbance; this can continue as a chronic problem.

- Subacute; this can be intermittent and only portrayed when the dog is tired, when it gets up in the morning, or after exercise and rest. The lifting of one leg can also occur with this.

The kyphotic dog, especially if in a chronic phase, can quite often be overlooked by the handler due to the slow progression of the condition, and because the various symptoms associated with the condition are easily ascribed to old age. Another typical example is a performance dog is lacking its former ability, or is habitually 'measuring' before a jump (a stuttering or shortening of stride in front of the jump, as if it has measured its stride incorrectly and is having to make adjustments) that is not typical behaviour.

Banana shape

This, too, can fit within any category, but it is generally seen in the acute phase, as it is often accompanied by a lack of weightbearing by one or other pelvic limb. This can also give the impression of a ligament problem. It, surprisingly, can be very easily missed, as assessing the dorsal aspect of a dog is not usually done; also, it is not easy for a very nervous dog to stand still long enough for the practitioner to make an accurate observation. This shape can cause shortening of the back on either side. Again, this is generally a deep lumbar issue, and it can be caused by action that results in extreme abduction or hyperextension of the coxofemoral joint. Figure **161** shows a mild case that only displayed a slight lack of weightbearing in one of the pelvic limbs.

Pelvic slide

This must be viewed with a degree of breed knowledge. A German Shepherd dog (GSD), or GSD cross, will probably have what could be defined as an accentuated angulation of the pelvis; however, this is normal for the breed, and is not the intended meaning of this pathological appearance. It is generally chronic, and the beginning of this condition can be traced back many months or years. The shape can produce a very poor gait that displays no flow or fluidity, with a very limited range of movement in the pelvic region. The pelvic muscles just 'fall away'; the dog is bearing weight behind through the hocks and stifles not the pelvis (**162**). A dog with this shape usually becomes 'torpedo'-shaped as drive from the pelvic region gradually diminishes.

The misfit

As the name implies, this is when there is a complete lack of congruence between the size and shape of the two sides, individual muscles, or muscle groups. This includes dogs that, in vehicular terms, may be described as 'cut and shut', i.e. the front end does not match the back end.

Weightbearing

This is an observation of how the dog stands. It can be the most revealing of the assessments. A dog should be weightbearing equally through each 'corner'; therefore, each foot should have the same area of pad on the ground, and there should be the same amount of flexion or extension of each joint in all four legs.

The therapist should consider whether comfort is displayed in the stand, or if there is 'paddling', a change of weightbearing by shuffling or subtle movements. Some dogs are trained so precisely to stand squarely, that this, coupled with their constant desire to please, means it is sometimes only the slightest of movements that differentiate between a comfortable or an uncomfortable stance. Weightbearing is most easily assessed by standing the dog on a flat hard surface and viewing it from behind, looking at the amount of weight that is being taken by the metatarsal and metacarpal pads of all of the legs. However, this can be difficult when the dog has hairy feet!

A good test for the assessment of balance is the diagonal hold (**164** *overleaf*). A perfectly balanced dog should be able to stand on two diagonally opposite legs without wobbling. When this test is performed, it is surprising how a dog showing very little imbalance (or, indeed, lameness) can be seen to be completely unbalanced. This test can indicate which of the diagonals is the weaker, and will help to locate the problem area further. This is also a good way to check the progress of treatment. Very occasionally, a dog may be equally wobbly on both diagonals.

During this exercise, the placement of the dog's feet should be observed (165): do they point medially or laterally? Do the front feet match? Do the back feet match? Do the nails have equal wear? Are the phalanges relaxed or tight, as if it were standing on tiptoe?

Weightbearing is not just assessed at the stand, it should be observed at the 'sit' and 'down' positions. The 'puppy sit' is generally not acceptable in a mature dog. If the dog shows an inclination to sit or lie to one side, this may be considered to be due to a problem that is worth investigating.

The 'look in the eye'

This can give psychological rather than physiological information, and pain perception may be reflected in the dog's look. The 'dead behind the eye' look is disturbing and can be difficult for the handler to interpret (166). However, some suggest that the dog does not react to pain in the same way as humans. Nevertheless, although this is subjective, a change in the 'look in the eye' may be apparent after treatment, when the pain has been eased (167).

Treatment

The torpedo

Typically, the source of the problem is in the pelvic region. The dog has had to compensate for pelvic problems and has developed 'front wheel drive' to assist its mobility, thereby completely changing its kinetic chain resulting in lameness in the thoracic limbs, or pain detected in the cervical region.

Dogs with this condition can develop massively hypertonic necks, recruiting all the dorsal/ventral flexion and extension muscles, plus all of the lateral flexion group. The neck hypertonicity can gravitate to the occipital region and to the m. frontalis, which develops heat and tension. This can give symptoms similar to a human having a headache: being

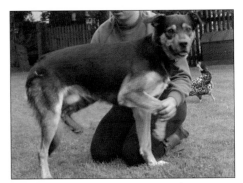

164 Lifting diagonally opposite feet is a good assessment tool of approximate total balance.

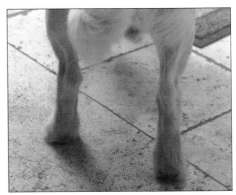

165 Observation of the hind feet in the assessment of weightbearing when standing.

depressed, craving darkened corners, and being photosensitive. The shoulder region will be involved, with the likelihood of hypersensitivity in the dorsomedial borders of the scapulae and caudal section of the m. trapezius, probably bilaterally. The m. brachiocephalicus (m. cleidocephalicus and m. cleidobrachialis) is painful during retraction of the thoracic limb. The pelvic area becomes hypotonic and weak due to lack of appropriate use. This is seen in all groups of dogs, but mostly in companion dogs, where minor pelvic injuries have perhaps not been picked up so quickly as in other groups. Microtrauma, and the slow but sustained accumulation of scar tissue result in reduced function of the muscle fibres in the pelvic region (**168, 169**).

A programme of intensive shoulder and neck therapy, together with passive movement, should be introduced. There should also be physical therapy to assist pelvic muscular and lumbar development.

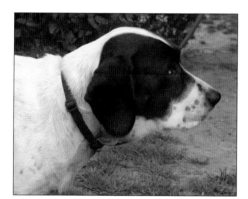
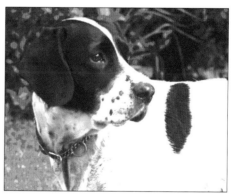

166, 167 Changes in the 'look behind the eyes' before (**166**) and after (**167**) three treatments.

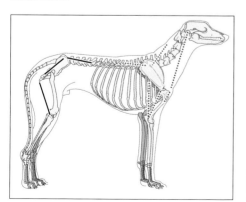
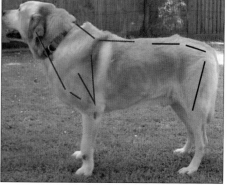

168, 169 Muscles affected by the torpedo shape. Black: hypotonic; red: hypertonic.

Half moon

This is a deep lumbar problem, with massive shortening of m. psoas, m. iliacus, and m. quadratus laborum. There is stretching of the gluteals and atrophy in m. rectus abdominus; this causes the transverse abdominal and external oblique muscles to be hypertrophic. Again, due to the lack of pelvic drive, there will be shoulder involvement, too. This is particularly seen in agility, flyball, and companion dogs with underlying problems such as undiagnosed cruciate disease, osteoarthritis, or subluxating patellas.

Passive movement should be used, easing the lumbar and gluteal regions. At times when the condition is not too severe, the addition of resistive exercise, e.g. hydrotherapy, may be helpful (**170, 171**).

Banana

If this is caught as early as the example in Figure **161**, the compensatory effects can be reduced, and the initial problem can be kept to a minimum, with unilateral involvement of m. psoas major, m. iliacus, and m. quadratus laborum (**172, 173**). However, if it is left untreated for some time, the other hip flexors, especially the quadricep group and m. tensor fascia latae will become involved, greatly affecting the dog's range of movement and flexibility.

This is seen in all groups, generally caused by a torque injury at speed, and usually because of a lack of core and general stability.

The hip flexors should be rebalanced and passive movement should be used. Resistive exercises, e.g. hydrotherapy, are indicated, as are core stability strengthening techniques.

Pelvic slide

Figures **174** and **175** depict a typical 'pelvic slide' shape and the problems this type of shape will present. Due to the stress caused from the shortening of the hamstring group of muscles there will be massive pivotal pressure in the pelvis, causing all of the intrinsic and extrinsic soft tissue to be involved. In response to the shortening of the hamstring group, some muscles will be constantly stretched: the quadricep group, mm. sartorius, and m. tensor fascia latae; this will also cause stress over the cranial aspect of the stifle. Stress develops at the thoraco-lumbar junction as a result of stress in the

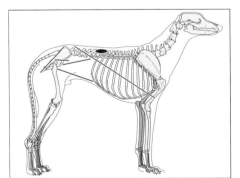
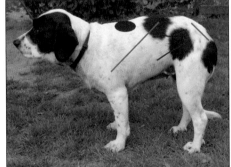

170, 171 Muscles affected by the half-moon shape. Blue: hypotonic muscles; red: hypertonic. The red circle represents the typical 'heat' point or stress point.

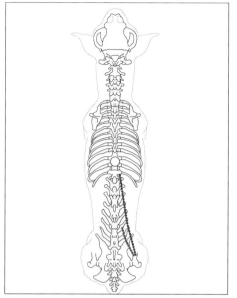 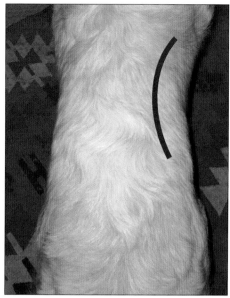

172, 173 Muscles involved in the banana shape. Red circle: stress point.

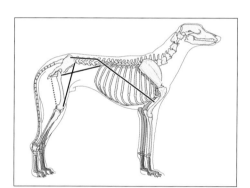 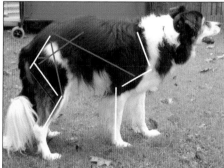

174,175 Muscles affected in pelvic slide. Blue; hypotonic; red: hypertonic; white: joint angulation.

mm. iliopsoas on both sides. The m. latissimus dorsi will also be involved, drawing fascially-related stress through from the pelvic region to the humerus, involving the thoracic region and reducing the range of movement. Due to compromised drive from the pelvic region, the thoracic region will be required to provide the forward motion, but it is already compromised. This is mainly seen in obedience and agility dogs. Contracture of the m. gracilis can look similar; this is most common in the GSD.

These dogs are typically in a great deal of pain due to the stresses and counter-stresses put on their skeletons. An easing of the shortened muscles will assist the pressure put on the whole body. This takes time, with good handler participation and continuing basic effleurage at home in order to ease and soothe the nerve endings and to assist vascular exchange, thereby enhancing muscular repair. Physical therapy can commence when the issue is no longer acute.

The misfit

By definition, this type of dog looks as if one end does not match the other, and there seems to be a definite dividing line between the two regions. A lack of stability between the thoracic and pelvic regions can be due to a variety of myofascial issues; a unilateral fascial tear at the myofascial junction of the m. latissimus dorsi is a possible cause. There can also be a deep pelvic problem surrounding the ligaments, but there is also a lack of hip flexor or stifle stability, manifested as a lack of good medial gluteal support. It may just be a result of poor conformation. This is particularly seen in dogs with poor core strength. All groups may be affected, but it is especially seen in the more lively breeds, or dogs that have been over-trained or allowed over-exertion from a young age.

Treatment varies according to the original problem.

Contraindications for canine massage

Massage is contraindicated in situations where using the therapy may cause further injury or exacerbate the existing condition. There are two key tenets that should always be remembered by therapists: Do no harm; if you are in any doubt, don't.

With those statements in mind, there are additional crucial factors to remember. Practitioners are offering secondary care; therefore, it is important to ensure that the dog has first been given a health check by a veterinary surgeon.

Due to many misconceptions, it is stated too many times that it 'can't do any harm'. That in itself is a potentially harmful statement! As stated previously, massage works on a very deep holistic cellular level, meaning that a topical treatment can be felt far beyond the point of application; thus, massage will influence many body systems. It cannot be stated strongly enough that the advantages and disadvantages of the use of massage must be properly considered before treatment is started. The first and most important precursor is to gain veterinary approval, consent, or referral. Not having this would be a contraindication.

Categories of contraindication

Some contraindications are absolute, when a dog is in such a poor physical state that any type of manipulative intervention that affects the body's healing processes and the reinstatement of homeostasis would be harmful, e.g. clinical shock or dehydration. Other contraindications are relative, meaning that the patient is at higher risk of complications than others, but that these risks may be outweighed by the potential pain relief offered by the treatment, e.g. in some forms of cancer. Some relative contraindications may also be of a local nature, where a particular area should be avoided, e.g. directly over a wound in its early stages of healing. Finally, some contraindications can be considered to be environmental, meaning when massage would be inappropriate in a normal healthy dog, e.g. just before or just after eating.

However, whatever the situation, massage is not a substitute for veterinary care.

To formulate a full list of contraindications is not possible, as it would not be definitive; *Tables 16–18* are merely a guide to the typical situations in which massage is contraindicated. As all cases will have veterinary consent, any questions about treatment and its suitability must be discussed with a veterinary surgeon.

Table 16 Absolute contraindications for massage

Situation	Explanation
Without veterinary approval, consent, or referral	Without an appropriate veterinary health check, underlying health conditions may not be known about, e.g. heart or circulatory conditions such as low blood pressure, anaemia, and so on
Clinical shock or fatigue	This can be a condition that can arise after an accident or when the dog has been, or still is, extremely stressed. In this case, the body 'switches off' and concentrates on maintaining the core organs: the brain, the heart, and so on. Massage would deflect heat and energy from these sites
Fever and infection (local or general)	The immune system will be working to resolve and nullify the effects of the condition and needs to do this without manipulative intervention that could prevent a natural healing process
Immediately after an accident or injury, or if a serious injury is suspected	Without any knowledge as to the extent of the injury and possible internal bruising or haemorrhage, more damage can easily be caused
Any form of undiagnosed pain	Without knowing the cause, more injury, or worsening of the condition, can be the result
Over an open wound, bruising, or oedema	Apart from the risk of causing pain or infection, massage would hinder healing
Over a lump (diagnosed or undiagnosed)	There is a risk of causing spread of a cancerous tumour by the encouragement of increasing the blood supply
If a dog is in any way unwell, or indicating an uncharacteristic dislike for touch or massage	There may be an underlying condition that would be contraindicative
Undiagnosed acute or chronic pain, e.g. spinal disc disease	Without any knowledge as to the extent of the injury or condition, serious damage can easily be caused

Table 17 Relative contraindications for massage

Situation	Explanation
In some types of cancer	Depending on the type of cancer, the risk of metastases can be the deciding factor when evaluating the potential beneficial effects of massage
Skin conditions	This depends on the condition: whether or not it can be spread through touch. If the cause is known, if it is not contagious, and if touch does not cause any discomfort, massage can be used as an aid to ease symptoms
Some post-operative cases	This depends on the type of operation. Professional advice must be sought
Some heart conditions	Different heart and circulatory conditions present with different symptoms: massage may be helpful for some, but not all. Professional advice must be sought

Table 18 Environmental contraindications for massage

Situation	Explanation
Immediately before being fed or less than 2 hours after treatment	The dog needs to be relaxed before eating. Thus, it should be in the correct neurological state for eating. Because the digestive system requires an enhanced blood supply to digest food successfully, massage will interfere with this process and will redirect the blood towards the muscles, possibly causing serious digestive problems. Also, massage should be avoided if the dog has just had head, neck, or jaw work
After strenuous exercise	The body needs to regain homeostasis; wait until the dog has resumed normal breathing
If the dog is excessively cold, hot, thirsty, or hungry	The body needs to regain homeostasis

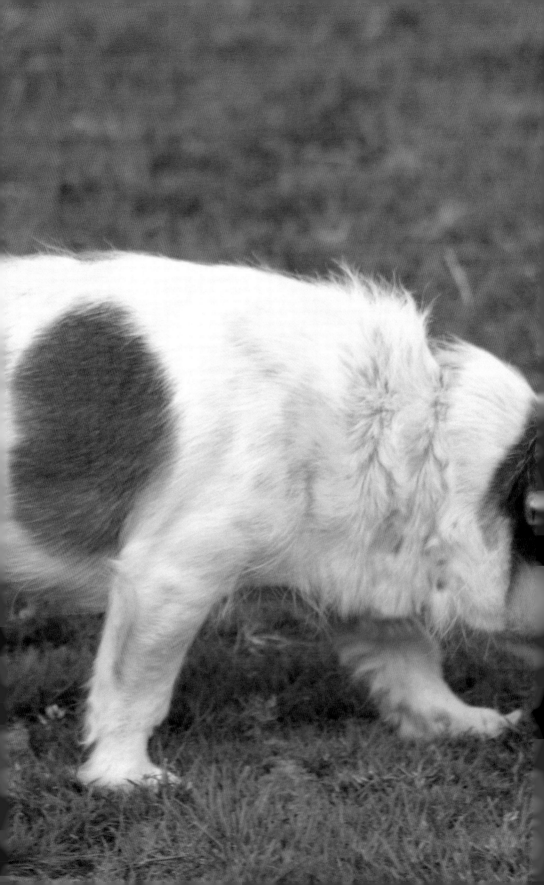

7

Common Diseases and Pathologies

Andy Mead and Julia Robertson

- Investigation of canine lameness
- Common joint diseases causing lameness
- Disorders of muscles and tendons
- Neoplasia
- Spinal disease
- Peripheral neurological disease

Investigation of canine lameness

The diagnosis of any lameness often presents a challenge. Diagnosis must be made by a qualified veterinary surgeon who, if unsure, will refer the case to an orthopaedic specialist. It is preferable that the primary cause of the lameness can be diagnosed and treated as early as possible in the disease process, as this will result in a more favourable prognosis. It is easier to make a diagnosis if the disease is more advanced, but this makes it more difficult to treat, and this will lead to a poorer prognosis.

Taking the history

One of the most important parts of the consultation and diagnostic process is taking a thorough history; this will precede the examination, which is also very important. This is true for both veterinarian and physiotherapist alike.

The following questions should be put to the handler in order to obtain a thorough and accurate signalment and history:

- What is the dog's signalment (age, breed, and sex)?
- How long has the owner owned the dog?
- How long have the clinical signs been present?
- Was there any traumatic event associated with the onset of lameness?
- Which limb or limbs are affected?
- Is the lameness worse at a particular time of day?
- Is it worse at particular times of year or in certain weather?
- Is there any change before or after exercise?
- Has the owner given any medication, or joint supplements, and did they help?
- Have any previous diagnoses been made?

The examination

In a case of lameness, the dog should be observed from afar to confirm the nature of the lameness, its severity, and to look for swelling, symmetry, or any obvious pathology. It is important that the clinician remains open-minded at this stage, as the owner's perception of lameness cannot be guaranteed to be correct, nor should it be assumed to be complete. Also, the veterinarian must be careful to avoid focusing in on the obvious and miss the less obvious problems. If time allows, the patient should be observed in motion, if possible at the walk and trot, over different surfaces (both hard and soft ground), coming towards and going away from the observer, and moving on a circle. This approach is adopted from the world of equine medicine, to give clues as to the likely position of the lameness of a horse. Lameness that worsens on hard or uneven ground may be indicative of the site of lameness being in the distal limb, whereas lameness that is worse on soft ground is more likely to be due to proximal limb problems, as the dog has to increase the range of motion of the upper limb.

Next, the whole of the dog is examined, but special attention is given to palpation of the affected limb/s. Palpation is possibly the single most important part of the physical examination of the dog. Touch provides information regarding heat, pain, swelling, joint effusion, and any notable differences between left and right. Thus, 'normal' anatomical features of the patient can be ruled out from being the cause of the pathology. Flexion and extension of the joints of the affected limb/s should be conducted, bearing in mind it is impossible to isolate all of the joints completely, such as the elbow and shoulder. Flexion of the elbow would result in some flexion of the shoulder, making it difficult to localize the affected area. Care should be taken, as the aim is not to exacerbate the condition, nor should the patient be aggravated. It should be remembered that different dogs will manifest discomfort in different ways. Salivation, a sideways glance, shifting weight onto different limbs, vocalizing, and obvious shows of aggression can all be indicative of pain.

Information gathered from the signalment (age, breed, and sex), history, and clinical examination can then be pieced together in order to form a tentative diagnosis, to direct further diagnostic procedures to confirm the suspected diagnosis, or to assist the commencement of appropriate therapy.

Diagnostic techniques

Sedation

It may be impossible to examine the fully conscious patient properly, due to the nature of the condition, or the inability to convince the patient to relax! Often, veterinarians will enlist the help of sedative drugs, or even induce general anaesthesia in order to fully manipulate the limbs and joints. This allows a more thorough examination of the dog, and removes the inherent stabilization of joints provided by the larger muscle groups. One example of a technique of manipulation that is attempted in the conscious patient, but which is more reliable if it is anaesthetized, is the cranial drawer test, a test to measure the congruity of the cranial/anterior cruciate ligament of the stifle (**176, 177**). Anterior and posterior movement of the tibia with respect to the femur is diagnostic of anterior cruciate ligament injury.

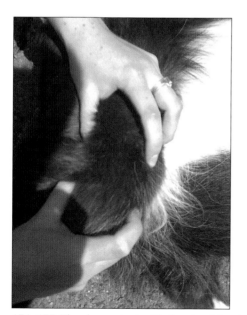
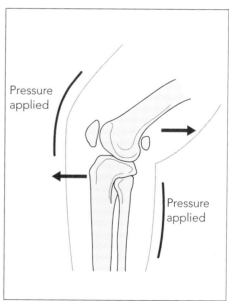

176, 177 The drawer test; with the dog lying in lateral recumbency, the hands grip the femur and tibia at the stifle. The tibia is slid cranially and caudally relative to the femur. (Arrows show direction of forces applied.)

Radiography

The most commonly used diagnostic technique in private practice is radiography. Radiography relies upon the generation of X-rays, a form of electromagnetic radiation, and the phenomenon by which they are absorbed by the structures of the body at varying rates. The electrons that are not absorbed hit the photographic plate placed behind the desired object and turn the photographic film from white to black. The image (radiograph or 'X-ray') is then developed much like a photograph, or converted to a computer-generated image (**178**).

Radiographs provide excellent images of the bony structures of the body, but offer little assistance in the diagnosis of soft tissue injury, due to the fact that bones absorb high levels of the electromagnetic radiation and soft tissue structures do not. Therefore, all soft tissues appear grey if they appear at all on a radiograph, depending on the exposure. However, bony structures appear white and are, therefore, clearly visible. One may uncover lesions that do not seem to relate to the lameness. In such situations, these should be assessed in relation to the clinical signs of disease in order to determine their significance. Accurate positioning and the application of the correct exposure are vital if one is to obtain radiographs of diagnostic quality, although, to a degree, this has been reduced by the advent of digital radiographic imaging software.

Further imaging techniques

More technologically advanced imaging techniques are becoming more widely available to aid in the diagnosis of lameness. Although they are expensive at the moment, it is widely accepted that these techniques will become more accessible in time.

Computed tomography

Computed tomography (CT) is similar to standard radiography save for the fact that several radiographs are made of slices of tissue in a particular region of the body in order to generate a computerized three-dimensional image. The major difference to radiography, however, is that soft tissues can be differentiated and examined far better with CT scans than with conventional radiography. Nevertheless, in cases of lameness, CT scans are best employed to examine bony structures of the body in finer detail.

Magnetic resonance imaging

Magnetic resonance imaging (MRI) involves the use of a very large magnetic field and radio waves to form images, which show very good soft tissue detail. As with CT, thin slices of tissue are imaged. MRI scans are of particular relevance when injury to soft tissue is suspected, e.g. muscle, tendon, or ligament. By taking images of several closely opposed slices of a particular joint, limb, muscle, or area, the images generated can be analysed in great detail, allowing even the most minute abnormalities to be detected. Furthermore, both CT and MRI provide a significant advantage to radiography in the evaluation of structures that are superimposed.

Ultrasonography

This is only occasionally used in a canine lameness work-up; its use is restricted due to the small size of dogs, and therefore the high resolution that is required. Within the equine world, ultrasonic scanning of tendons is considered routine.

Piezo-electric crystals contained within a probe emit ultrasonic waves that can pass through most structures apart from bone, before being reflected back to the probe (**179**). The wavelength of these ultrasonic beams can be altered to increase the penetration of the wave, with lower frequencies travelling further than higher frequency waves. Also, the wavelength should be reduced to provide a more detailed image but without penetrating deep structures. As joints tend to be close

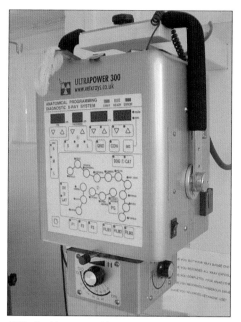

178 An X-ray machine.

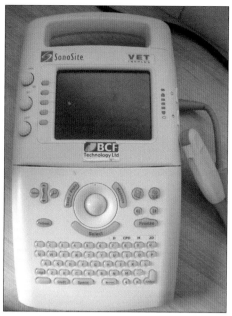

179 Ultrasound scanner and probe (5–10 MHz) typically available in general veterinary practice.

to the surface of the body, with little soft tissue coverage, very high-frequency probes would be required to produce images of diagnostic quality in cases of lameness. These are expensive and, therefore, rarely available to the general practitioner.

Arthroscopy
Small cameras can be placed into joints to examine their interior surfaces, through small incisions known as 'keyholes'. Damaged cartilage is often removed or repaired at the same time through these incisions. Arthroscopy is an extremely valuable tool when investigating lesions identified by radiography further, in order to ascertain their significance.

Further diagnostic techniques
Arthrocentesis

Arthrocentesis is often performed along with radiography, under a single anaesthetic. The technique involves the aseptic placement of a needle into the joint. Samples of the joint fluid are collected in various containers for microscopic examination and/or bacterial culture, in order to provide information regarding the cause of the joint disease, but it is also examined by eye and touch first to observe the quality, viscosity, and quantity of the joint fluid. The molecular weights of the compounds present within the fluid can also be analysed. It is a relatively simple procedure to perform, and not only provides information regarding the disease process, but also the efficacy of treatments given (180).

Common joint diseases causing lameness

Osteoarthritis (OA) (arthritis, degenerative joint disease [DJD], secondary joint disease)

Arthritis is the inflammation of a joint; there are, however, over 100 types, depending on the cause, including bacterial, degenerative, enteropathic (associated with bowel disease), neonatal, rheumatoid, septic, and traumatic. The word 'osteoarthritis' is derived from the Greek osteo, meaning 'of the bone', arthro, meaning 'joint', and itis, meaning 'inflammation'. OA is the end stage of several disease processes, and each name used has different merits. DJD is a particularly descriptive term, suggestive of

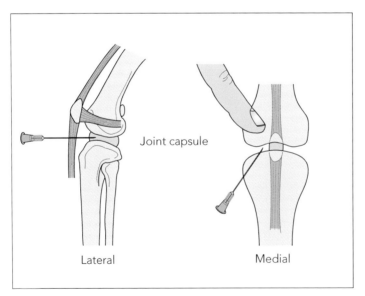

180 Arthrocentesis technique for the canine stifle.

Joint capsule

Lateral

Medial

deterioration, or change to a less functional form. The term does not discriminate between different ages or species. The suggestion is, however, of an end-stage condition; this term best represents the latter stages of a collection of joint diseases.

OA is defined as a 'noninflammatory degenerative joint disease marked by degeneration of the articular cartilage, hypertrophy/sclerosis of the bone at the margins of the joint, and changes in the synovialmembrane'. This seems somewhat contradictory. Such definitions cause intense debate, as it is widely accepted that in the early stages of the disease, inflammation certainly plays a critical role in producing the clinical signs of joint pain, and reducing the inflammation seems to be a crucial part of its treatment. It is implied, therefore, that the term OA is more suggestive of the chronicity of the disease. Indeed, pro-inflammatory cytokines (mediators of inflammation) have been found in high numbers within joints, and these contribute to OA and inflammation. In contrast, another less commonly used term, 'secondary joint disease' implies that the inflammation/joint disease has occurred as a result of a predisposing issue or has derived from a previous condition. This term has restricted use today, however. For the purposes of this text, the terms OA and DJD will be used.

DJD is one of the oldest diseases known to man, evidence of the disease having been found in the fossilized remains of early dinosaurs. It is also all too common, accounting for the vast majority of cases of arthritis in both dogs and humans, and, indeed, it has become one of the most prevalent and disabling chronic diseases.

DJD results in the loss of substances called proteoglycans or glycoproteins, which consist of chains of complex sugar molecules all linked to an amino acid molecule, amino acids being the building blocks of protein. The loss of proteoglycans from the articular cartilage collagen matrix causes weakening and it becoming brittle. As a result, the cartilage becomes less elastic, leading to fissuring. When a joint is loaded, some of the water from the matrix is squeezed out of the articular cartilage, thereby reducing friction and, it is proposed, providing nutrition to the surface of the cartilage. If the proteoglycans structure is altered, the attractiveness to water (via osmosis) will be reduced. Consequently, not only is the structure of the cartilage weakened, but it also becomes less rigid. The friction in the joint is increased, further destroying the cartilage in what becomes a vicious cycle. The destruction of glycoproteins and increase of friction forces within the joint lead to destruction of the synovium, a thin layer of cells dedicated to joint fluid production. Therefore, the affected joint suffers not only from increased friction, but also from a reduction in joint fluid required to reduce its effects.

The mechanism by which new bone is laid down at the articular margins is not well understood. However, it is surmised that osteocytes, bone-producing cells, are stimulated by damage of the articular cartilage, leading to an inflammatory cascade. Movement of the joint exacerbates the development of new bone around the margins, and therefore the deposits become more pronounced. It could be considered that the body is attempting to fuse, or arthrodese, the joint in question in order to reduce pain and friction associated with the degenerative process. In summary, the pathological changes associated with OA include cartilage loss, sclerosis, or thickening, of bone directly adjacent to the joint, new bone formation at the margins of the joint, and inflammation of the synovium (181, 182).

As a general rule, patients with OA/DJD will have a long history of insidious lameness, possibly exacerbated by sudden trauma or by a particularly long walk on the preceding day. However, the progression of OA is variable, some cases remaining subclinical for many years.

The predominant causes of DJD include trauma, leading to malformation of a joint, wear and tear, congenital deformities that predispose an animal to abnormal wear and tear, cartilage malformation, nutritional deficiencies, growth abnormalities, infection, immune-mediated disease, and neoplasia or tumours. Several of the most common causes will be discussed in detail subsequently. Fundamentally, all of the above will result in instability of the joint and, therefore, abnormal movement. OA should not be confused with other, rarer forms of arthritis which also lead to DJD. These include septic arthritis (infection) and rheumatoid arthritis (an immune-mediated condition). Fortunately, both are extremely rarely diagnosed in animals. The upshot of the degenerative process is that the animal begins to feel pain (presumably due to the fissuring of the articular surface setting off an inflammatory reaction) when manipulating the joint, or during normal movement, and shows progressive stiffness, leading to the exhibition of an awkward gait. With time and progression just rising or standing can become exceedingly painful for the sufferer.

The impact of DJD is not usually restricted to just one joint. Even if it were, it is only natural that if a particular joint becomes painful, every attempt would be made, either consciously or subconsciously, to reduce friction in that joint by reducing its movement. Extra strain will

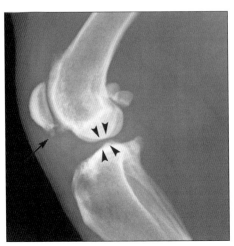

181 Radiograph of a dog's stifle with OA. Note the irregular periosteal new bone (arrow) and subchondral sclerosis (arrowheads).

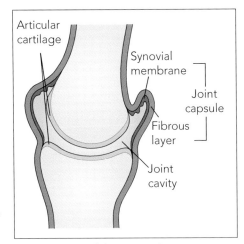

182 Diagram of the synovial joint.

therefore be placed upon adjacent muscles, ligaments, and tendons, for which they were not designed, leading to further destabilization. Decreased movement of a joint will in time lead to associated muscle atrophy, further compounding the problem by reducing even further the ability of the joint to undergo its normal function. This is where the canine physiotherapist can undoubtedly make a significant difference by keeping the joints supple, reducing associated muscle atrophy, and maintaining, as much as possible, normal use of a joint.

Radiographic changes that occur with DJD (or with any skeletal pathology) will vary from patient to patient and with stage of disease. Radiographic signs of DJD include the presence of periosteal new bone at the articular margins, subchondral sclerosis (thickening of the bone around the joints, appearing as more whiteness), cartilage loss, joint effusion, or reduction in the size of the joint space.

Common causes of OA/DJD

Developmental arthropathies such as elbow or hip dysplasia, as well as those that are acquired, for example articular fractures or ligament injuries, can instigate the degenerative process of OA. To some extent, causes of OA/DJD are inter-related, but for clarity will be discussed separately below.

Excessive weight and uneven exercise schedules

It is not difficult to see that obviously overweight dogs will place undue and excess strain on joints and muscles, leading to OA, so weight should be reduced where possible.

Exercise modification should also be instigated, if appropriate, as OA may be caused or exacerbated by excessive exercise. Unfortunately, modern life tends to dictate that dogs receive short walks during the busy working week, then long walks at weekends as part of our relaxation process. This may be a contributory factor in the development of OA, and will aggravate it if it has already begun (see Chapter 4). Would a footballer train for 5 minutes a day during the week to play for 90 on a Saturday? If DJD has already set in, long walks will become unnecessarily painful and cause further deterioration by increasing abnormal wear and tear on already compromised joints.

Trauma

Trauma is considered to be the most common cause of OA/DJD. A traumatic incident can be severe, causing a fracture of the joint leading to healing which will probably cause malformation of that joint surface, or very minor, but frequent and cumulative in the case of chronic, repetitive wear and tear. Age has also been blamed, some believing that age-related changes to the cartilage are responsible for the arthritis observed. Certainly, it has been shown that the joint space and the water content of the cartilage reduce in later life. It is important to reiterate that anything that causes a joint to become unstable, thereby affecting the way by which forces are dissipated within the joint, could arguably be deemed to have an involvement in the development of OA, no matter how innocuous it seems at the time.

Wear and tear

The process of wear and tear is poorly understood in this context. However, it is completely logical, similar to needing to replace the tyres or brakes on a car from time to time. Two schools of thought exist: one suggests that irritant chemicals are released from the cartilage, causing damage to surrounding tissue and instigating OA; the second suggests that the constant trauma to joints as a result of being mechanically loaded and then unloaded causes damage.

Conformational abnormalities

Abnormal conformation of joints will undoubtedly lead to abnormal use and, therefore, abnormal wear and tear. Any joint is severely affected by alterations, however minor, in the forces that are spread across its surfaces, and any abnormal destruction or deterioration in the cartilage of the articular surface that results will lead to OA.

Growth plate trauma
Growth and development of the long bones has been discussed in detail previously. Endochondral ossification occurs predominantly at the metaphyseal growth plate (see Chapter 2). Only when the growth plates cannot be detected radiographically can an animal be considered skeletally mature (see Chapter 3) (*Table 19*). Trauma to this region during the growing process can be devastating, leading to limb deformities. These may, in future, predispose the animal to OA as a consequence of abnormal load bearing.

Juvenile cancellous bone is inherently weak and, therefore, trauma is usually more destructive than in the adult. However, the properties of juvenile periosteum, which is both thick and strong, provide a further source of growth and stability should growth plates be traumatized.

Treatment modalities
The treatment of OA/DJD relies, firstly, on the treatment of any underlying cause, if possible. This must be done in order to prevent further deterioration of a joint; for

Table 19 Average times of closure of selected growth plates

Long bone	Growth plate	Age at radiographic closure (months)
Femur	Femoral head	10.5
	Greater trochanter	10.5
	Distal	11
Humerus	Proximal	12.5
	Lateral condyle	6
Radius	Proximal	11
Tibia	Proximal	11

Adapted from BSAVA Manual of Small Animal Fracture Repair and Management (Coughlan and Miller, 1998).

example, repair of a ruptured cruciate ligament must be done in order to prevent further joint instability and DJD. Often, it is the aim of the veterinary surgeon to manage the condition rather than to cure it, as, by the time of diagnosis, the degeneration of a joint/s is already significant. Any treatment regime should not be directed solely at the treatment of pain and inflammation, or at the increase of joint fluid production, but aimed at the reduction of severity of clinical signs, attaining an improvement in animal welfare, and the prevention of further deterioration of the condition. To this end, treatment is often multi-factorial; medical and surgical treatments are employed both separately and in combination, and also in association with physiotherapy and hydrotherapy.

Weight and exercise

These have been mentioned previously; they are very common underlying causes of DJD, and should be addressed as soon as possible. However, all too often, these factors fail to be considered when a treatment protocol is designed.

It is believed that regular lead exercise is preferable, as this will help the dog to remain mobile; well-conditioned muscle and good muscular balance are important factors in the attenuation of the impact load. However, jumping, climbing, and twisting, which will undoubtedly exacerbate clinical signs of OA, should be prevented, as these represent abnormal or excessive movements for affected joints.

Medical treatment

Anti-inflammatory and pain-relieving medication

Commercial, prescription-only (POM) and nonprescription medications (over-the-counter, OTC) for OA are widely available. Nonsteroidal anti-inflammatory drugs (NSAIDs) are arguably most commonly prescribed. NSAIDs such as meloxicam and carprofen target the inflammatory processes involved with OA, reducing cartilage degeneration, as well as reducing pain associated with synovial inflammation. Their efficacy is well documented. Any reduction in pain will allow for improved and more natural movement of a joint, bone, or muscle. NSAIDS exert their beneficial effects by inhibition of the enzymes COX 1 and COX 2 which prevent the formation of prostaglandins, the instigators of inflammation. The more modern NSAIDs preferentially block only one of these enzymes, thus the beneficial aspects of these enzymes (the generation of protective matrices for the bladder and stomach walls) is preserved. This property has made NSAIDs more popular than corticosteroids, which were once widely utilized, but long-term use of corticosteroids may cause serious side-effects, including gastric ulceration and the development of iatrogenic Cushing's disease. The effect of such products on synovial inflammation is thought to be small; improvement in demeanour and gait are probably more likely to be a result of their analgesic properties. Therefore, the role of an NSAID is to prevent the abnormal loading of joints by the promotion of normal joint activity.

The aim when using any such therapy is to use the lowest dose-rate possible to alleviate clinical signs, and, therefore, to minimize the risks of detrimental side-effects. Many preparations are currently licensed for the treatment of OA and for long-term use.

As with any veterinary prescription only medicine (POM-V), they must be given in accordance with veterinary instruction and supervision, entailing regular checkups and blood tests to monitor liver and kidney function. This ensures the animal is benefitting from the correct dosing regime and able to excrete the by-products safely and effectively.

Important note: please remember that many human pain killers, such as aspirin, paracetamol, and ibuprofen, are poisonous to dogs at human dose rates, and should never be administered.

Pentosan polysulphate

Another POM-V drug used in the treatment of OA in dogs is pentosan polysulphate (PPS). PPS has been developed to afford 'chondro-protection' rather than solely to relieve the clinical symptoms of arthritis. It is often used in conjunction with NSAIDs as part of a multi-drug approach to the long-term treatment of OA. The efficacy of PPS has been demonstrated in the dog when it is administered both orally and, in a separate study, subcutaneously. Its action is three-fold: it is believed to promote the synthesis of glycosaminoglycans necessary for joint lubrication, to act as an anticoagulant, and to down-regulate detrimental enzymes stimulated by inflammation and the degradation of cartilage within a joint.

Nutraceuticals

The use of 'nutraceutical' medications, both for the prophylaxis and treatment of OA has become more widespread in recent years. In the USA, one study reported that 30% of pet owners had used or considered using nutraceuticals for their animals. The belief held by many is that such products can do no harm, as they largely consist of naturally occurring substances and, therefore, such treatments appear more 'natural'. However, regulation of such medications is limited and, therefore, one should always use those from a reputable source. Examples commonly available include chondroitin sulphate and glucosamine.

The intended purpose of nutraceuticals is to provide nutrition to the synovial cells of the joint, to promote normal joint structure and function, and, in some cases, to decrease inflammation. Some act as free-radical scavengers, reducing damage to adjacent joint cells, and replacing or supplementing joint fluid. Their use is believed, in certain circumstances, to reduce the dose of NSAIDs, or even the need for their long-term usage at all.

Several preparations are available in the UK, with widely varying costs and therapeutic claims. Little proof of their efficacy has been established so far, however. Human trials measuring a reduction in joint space as an indicator of OA have, however, proved positive. Investigations into the efficacy of other popular treatments, including avocado, green-lipped mussel, soya bean, and so-called 'devil's claw', are ongoing.

Advances in the medical treatment of OA

Future treatment developments rely on targeting the processes involved in arthritis more specifically, for example, the inhibition of enzymes believed to cause cartilage destruction (so-called proteolytic enzymes). Also, future advances are likely to be better targeted at individual inflammatory mediators, for example, a group of enzymes called metallo-proteinases, found in high numbers within the chondrocytes of affected joints. These enzymes are believed to promote a catabolic state within the joint, and are potential targets for future therapy.

Surgical treatment

In certain circumstances, surgery to repair or replace an affected joint is considered. Procedures include femoral head and neck excision (see later), total hip replacement, and elbow replacement, as well as procedures to correct the underlying causes of OA, for example cruciate rupture and hip dysplasia (see later). It should be ensured, however, that a period of strict rest and rehabilitation can and must be undertaken after such surgical procedures. The negative effects of long periods of cage rest or exercise restriction should be outweighed by the amelioration or prevention of pain and discomfort. Temperament and age are often critical factors when making the decision whether to opt for surgical treatment.

Myotherapy /massage

Pain from secondary muscle problems, such as compensatory problems, can sometimes be as great as the arthritis itself. By easing the injured or shortened muscle that may have been involved in the original injury or trauma that surrounds the affected joint, or by lessening the tension distal to the area, can have a surprisingly fast effect on the dog from both physiological and psychological perspectives. This is one treatment area that can lead to vast improvements within the mobility and general wellbeing of the dog. This is especially important to dogs that are sensitive to NSAIDs, or those that will probably need protracted medical treatment.

Easing the stresses on the affected area, thereby instigating a change of muscle patterning and promoting a more normal gait, can lead to a holistic change within the dog, by redistributing muscle mass (see Chapter 6). A programme of initial treatments followed by a planned future treatment programme can be extremely successful, and can maintain mobility and, therefore, stabilize the condition in the long term.

Hip dysplasia

Hip dysplasia (HD) is a developmental disease, predominantly of large and giant breeds. The aetiology of HD is multifactorial, the major predisposing factor being joint laxity (looseness).

Canine HD inevitably leads to secondary DJD.

The processes that lead to DJD, with resultant lameness and discernibly altered gait, begin soon after birth. Environmental factors, such as rapid weight gain and excessive exercise, exacerbate the problem. At birth, hips appear macroscopically (to the eye) unaffected, but, as joint looseness or laxity worsens with age, the joint capsule and ligaments that attach the femoral head to the acetabulum become stretched. This leads to subluxation (partial dislocation) of the hip/s. From an early stage of the disease process, load and friction forces are applied to a weakened joint, forcing them to be dissipated in an abnormal manner. The disease process then progresses towards DJD, through various stages:

- Cartilaginous destruction and transformation from stiff gel to brittle noncompliant material.
- Erosion of joint margins.
- Sclerosis and bruising of subchondral bone.
- Pain.
- Bony remodelling, osteophyte production at articular margins, and widening of the joint surfaces to increase the load-bearing surface.
- Scarring of the joint capsule and formation of fibrous tissue.
- Reduction in joint laxity.

The process is, in part, the body's attempt to heal itself by stabilizing the joint. The intention is to reduce movement and, therefore, to reduce pain. This leads to a reduction in subsequent damage to the cartilage, synovial cells, and so on.

`Radiographically, the evidence is present even in the skeletally immature animal, but as the degenerative changes are cumulative, they become much more obvious with time (183, 184). The disease appears bilateral, but one limb may be predominantly affected, leading to exacerbated clinical signs in that limb. However, perhaps surprisingly, many dogs are asymptomatic clinically, and dysplasia is only diagnosed incidentally, prior to breeding or during diagnostic procedures for other diseases.

Veterinarians and physiotherapy practitioners tend to examine dogs suffering from HD when degeneration of muscles surrounding the hip has already occurred, and the ability of the dog to compensate for the instability of the joint is already greatly reduced. By this stage, the arthritic process is well under way; the disease is manifesting itself in pain and inflammation of the joints. This can occur in animals as young as 2 years old. Occasionally, dysplasia can be exhibited at an even earlier stage, when the teres ligament and joint capsule have become lax. Here, pain is unlikely to be due to arthritis, but is probably caused by the abnormal way in which weight is borne. Classically, during the movement of the worst cases, there is rotation of the hips, or an attempt to reduce extension of the hip joint, causing a wiggle similar to that of a catwalk model. Palpation may show substantial development of the supporting muscles of the hips, or, indeed, reduction in their mass, should the disease process be more advanced. Extension of the hip (185) elicits pain, often manifested by protective aggression. A reduced range of motion is also noted.

Treatment

To date, no cure has been described, so control is paramount. This relies upon the identification of genetic factors, and attempts to reduce the number and severity of cases by careful breeding of affected breeds. In sufferers, the

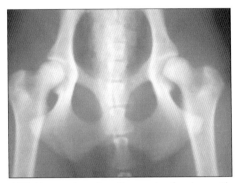

183 Ventrodorsal radiograph of a dog with minimal evidence of degenerative joint disease.

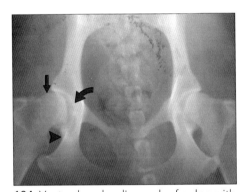

184 Ventrodorsal radiograph of a dog with advanced HD and DJD. Note the thickening of the femoral neck (arrow), the osteophyte formation (arrowhead), the flattening of the femoral head (curved arrow), and the reduction of the amount of the femoral head within the acetabulum.

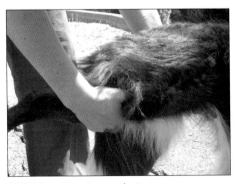

185 Hip extension technique.

CASE STUDY 5

Dexter, the German Shepherd dog: from hip dysplasia to Crufts 2006 winner

When Dexter was 18 months old, his owner, Kelly Lovebury, learned that his hip score was very high, indicating that he had bad HD. This could have spelled a very limited existence for Dexter, but Kelly had other ideas. In consultation with her vet, Kelly avoided giving him anti-inflammatory drugs, and hydrotherapy was chosen instead. Dexter responded well to this between the ages of 2 and 7 years, and improved sufficiently to begin training and competing in obedience trials. Unfortunately, once he reached 7 years old, he slowly started to change: his back became stiffer, and his turns became wider and much less balanced.

Kelly came to a talk given by Julia Robertson about the benefits of canine myotherapy and massage therapy, following which Kelly brought Dexter to the Galen Therapy Centre for assessment and treatment. Upon his arrival at the clinic, Julia noticed the unnatural roaching of his back which had evolved slowly over time. The massage therapy he received that day released muscular spasm and eased this. Further targeted treatments facilitated a change within Dexter's biomechanics, which resulted in altering the way he moved and which muscles he used. Dexter was also put on a programme of core-stability exercises, to further strengthen the deep pelvic muscles, enabling him to be more balanced, and, therefore, to build up the muscles supporting the badly formed joints. Within 2 months, the roaching had disappeared, and Dexter's balance had improved significantly. He continued to attend hydrotherapy sessions to support and build up his new muscle pattern.

Amazingly, in the spring of 2006, Dexter not only qualified for Crufts in the Kennel Club young handler obedience elementary class, but won against enormous competition in his class. The judge even complimented Kelly's daughter, Jessica, on his balance.

amelioration of clinical signs is important. Specific treatment options are available to the dysplastic patient, ranging from conservative to surgical. Conservative methods employed are similar to those used for any arthritic patient: they include the use of NSAIDs, nutraceuticals, physiotherapy, and hydrotherapy. Surgical options are available, but great care must be taken over case selection, and consideration given to the long recovery periods. Surgical treatments include total hip replacement, triple pelvic osteotomy, and femoral head and neck excision.

Despite the serious nature and early onset of the disease, with the correct treatment many dogs do have a good quality of life, and remain pain free. The genetic predisposition of certain breeds has led to schemes aimed at eradicating the problem, breeding animals being rigorously screened for the presence of congenital disease, and registration of puppies by the Kennel Club being declined should the parents either have poor hip conformation or if screening has not taken place.

Myotherapy/massage therapy

The sooner dogs with HD can receive muscle-balancing therapy, the sooner inappropriate stresses (piezo-electric changes) can be prevented. Like OA, this condition has to be managed from the day of diagnosis; this takes dedication, but the results can be surprisingly good.

Once HD has been diagnosed, myo-therapy can help to rebalance the muscular system, easing the compensatory muscle issues employed by the body to stabilize the coxofemoral joint. There needs to be a well-managed plan of limited exercise to ensure the slightly exposed joint is not compromised. During this time, a programme of pelvic postural muscle-balancing can commence, and this is something that can successfully be carried out by the handler at home (see Chapter 6). The concept is simple, but the results can be outstanding, especially if they start early after diagnosis. Once stability and appropriate muscular balance can be felt by the practitioner and also observed by the handler, hydrotherapy is highly beneficial. To help maintain the balance, the pelvic stability exercises and hydrotherapy should be continued with regular myotherapy sessions. Dexter's story underlines the success of these treatments.

Osteochondritis dissecans

Osteochondritis dissecans (OCD) is possibly one of the most common diseases affecting young dogs, and a major causal factor in the development of OA or DJD in later life. Osteochondrosis is defined as the failure of cartilage maturation within a joint, and occurs as a result of a disturbance of the process of endo-chondral ossification, described previously (see Chapter 2). By disturbing the maturation process, possibly due to the reduction of blood supply to the area, the cartilage of an affected joint becomes thickened, brittle (due to poor nutrition), and loses both its stiff, gel-like consistency and its ability to dissipate friction forces. The cartilage subsequently becomes prone to cracking; as a result, cartilage flaps form, and fragments (or joint mice), often microscopic in size, shatter off into the synovial space. Inevitably, this leads to an inflammatory response as the body tries to remove these, and also because the fissures form channels for inflammatory mediators to reach the joint (186). The inflammatory response is often considered to be over-exaggerated. Male dogs seem to be over-represented in studies of the disease leading to the postulation that there may be a hormonal input to the disease process. OCD affects medium and large breeds from 4 to 12 months of age, although many are diagnosed far later, when DJD develops. This highlights the need for the history and signalment to be taken into account during the diagnostic process.

Normally, affected dogs present with a unilateral lameness, despite the fact that the disease process invariably affects both limbs to some degree. Clinical signs do not appear until a cartilage flap has developed. Owners often describe their pets as being slow, unwilling to exercise, or that they have a change in their gait. In severe cases, lameness on rising or after periods of prolonged inactivity is observed.

The precise aetiology of OCD is unknown, but it is certain that nutrition and exercise have a significant role to play. It is this knowledge that has led to advice relating to the partial restriction of exercise in young maturing animals, and ensuring that overfeeding, leading to rapid growth, does not occur. It is important to reiterate the significance of growth plates during bone development, and their average times of closure (187) (see Chapter 2 and *Table 19*).

The most common site for OCD is the shoulder, with the elbow also being a frequently affected site (188, 189). Other predilection sites are the carpus, the foot, the hip, the stifle, and the hock. Often, radiographic changes are particularly subtle and are, therefore, difficult to detect by veterinary general practitioners using simple X-ray machines. With progression of the disease process, such lesions become far more obvious radiographically,

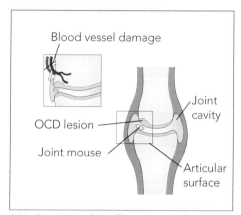

186 Diagram of a stifle joint with lesions due to OCD.

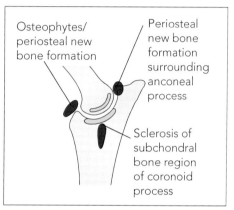

188 Diagram showing common sites of OCD in the elbow joint.

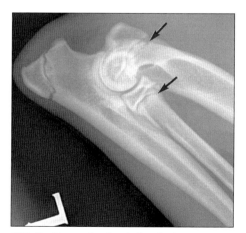

187 Radiograph of a skeletally immature dog showing open growth plates (arrows).

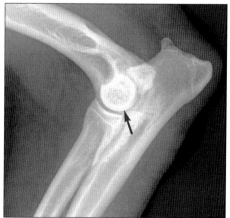

189 Lateral radiograph of the elbow showing OCD of the medial coronoid process (arrow).

as does clinical suspicion based upon clinical examination. Therefore, early detection is crucial, in order to prevent progression of the disease. Dogs with the correct signalment that are exhibiting clinical signs suggestive of OCD should be referred to larger veterinary centres, where more sensitive imaging modalities may aid in the diagnosis of OCD.

Treatment

Treatment of OCD is similar to that previously described for OA and, once again, it is aimed at reducing pain and inflammation, as well as promoting normal movement of the joint. Arthroscopy or surgery to repair or remove damaged cartilage is widely employed. Dietary and exercise modification appear to be critical in the prevention of the disease. The prognosis is usually good if the disease is caught early enough, prior to the development of secondary changes.

Panosteitis

The name suggests inflammation of both cortical and medullary bone, affecting bone marrow initially. Usually long bones of large breed, typically male dogs are affected, with new bone formation and remodelling particularly evident within the diaphysis (**190**). An increase in intramedullary density is noted after radiographic examination with indistinct margins. The radiographic changes can, however, be just as subtle as those of OCD, so the comments on the diagnosis of OCD also apply here.

It is a painful condition, possibly underdiagnosed, usually presenting with a history of a waxing and waning shifting lameness. Elevated temperatures are noted on physical examination, as well as a pain response on palpation of the long bones affected, usually elicited by gently squeezing the diaphysis. Often several bones are affected simultaneously or at different stages of the disease process, which is selflimiting.

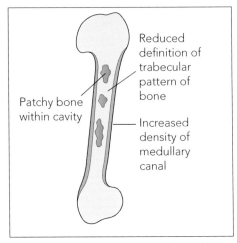

190 Diagram of a long bone affected by panosteitis.

Labels: Reduced definition of trabecular pattern of bone; Patchy bone within cavity; Increased density of medullary canal

Treatment

Again, there is no cure for panosteitis; management of the pain associated with the condition can, however, be helpful. Like all lameness issues, whether chronic or acute, the maintenance of muscular integrity and balance with myotherapy and massage can significantly reduce the pain and, more importantly, can treat any secondary conditions that may be caused through inappropriate stresses distal to the affected area.

Legg–Calvé–Perthes disease

Legg–Calvé–Perthes disease (LCPD) is a condition predominantly affecting small dogs, particularly West Highland White Terriers. It is, fundamentally, a specific form of OCD. Thankfully an uncommon degenerative arthropathy, its clinical symptoms are similar to those of HD, and include sudden or slow onset lameness, stiffness or pain on manipulation of the hip joint and, most noticeably, a reduction in the ability to extend the hip. Often one pelvic limb may appear shorter than the other. It is suggested that the aetiology of the disease is the reduction in blood supply to the femoral head and neck, leading to necrosis of cells through lack of nutrition and oxygen. As a consequence, changes similar to those of OA occur, particularly as the necrotic cells of the femoral head and neck are replaced by weaker fibrovascular tissue, leading to weakening of the normal structure of trabecular bone; as a result, this 'crumbles' with the traumatic forces applied when extending or adducting the hip. The precise cause of the damage to the blood supply to the epiphysis of the femur is unclear, but a hereditary cause is suspected.

Treatment

Conservative management, as described earlier, should be tried first. However, if this fails, surgical intervention is indicated: a femoral head and neck excision is performed. Here, the fibrosed head and neck of the femur is removed, reducing the contact between the femur and the acetabulum, thereby reducing pain and further degeneration of the region (191, 192). A fibrous joint is created as a result, which serves the animal well. Post-surgically, the joint remains unstable, and therefore the procedure should only be undertaken as a salvage procedure, where financial constraints mean that a total hip replacement is not a viable option.

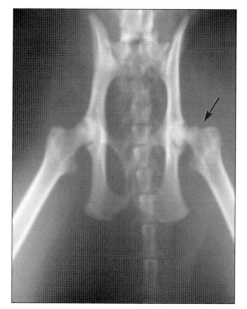

191 Ventrodorsal radiograph showing fracture of femoral head (arrow).

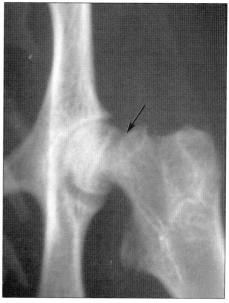

192 Close up of fracture line (arrow).

Post-surgically, this condition can be helped enormously by appropriate myotherapy, massage, and scar management. The sooner these begin after surgery, the more effective they are. The treatment is suited to the individual, but is similar to that for HD.

Septic arthritis

As the name suggests, this type of arthritis is caused by (usually bacterial) infection. The bacteria are often inoculated into a joint after trauma or the occurrence of a deep penetrating wound to a joint. Infection of post-surgical wounds and bacterial inoculations during arthrocentesis are common causes; hence, maximum sterility should be maintained whenever such procedures are undertaken.

Contamination of the joint with bacteria leads to the inevitable inflammatory response, the deposition of fibrin and white blood cells, and an increase in the fluid volume of the joint. In an attempt to eradicate the bacteria, enzymes released by the white blood cells damage the cartilage matrix and the synovial cells, impairing joint fluid production and nutrition of articular cartilage. The process is similar to that of any secondary joint disease.

Clinical symptoms and radiographic changes noted are similar to those of OA; therefore, the diagnosis can only be confirmed by arthrocentesis, followed by bacterial culture of the joint fluid. Bacterial arthritis may be strongly suspected if there is a history of direct trauma to a joint.

Noninfectious inflammatory joint disease

Rheumatoid arthritis and other forms of immune-mediated arthritis are rare in the dog. Essentially, in these conditions the joint surfaces are mistaken as foreign. As yet, no causal agent has been determined, but this condition initiates inflammatory pathways that inevitably lead to DJD.

Luxation of the patella

Patellar luxation involves displacement or dislocation of the patella from the trochlear groove. The patella, encapsulated by the patellar tendon, is able to move dorsally and ventrally, acting as a hinge to enable flexion and extension of the knee. Luxation allows side-to-side movement, which leads to lameness. It is common in small dogs, but should not be ignored as a cause of lameness amongst larger breeds. In general, the smaller breeds suffer a medial displacement, as opposed to large breeds, in which a lateral luxation of the patella occurs.

The patellar tendon is attached to the quadriceps muscle, and an underlying malalignment of the quadriceps muscle is often blamed for this developmental condition. The displaced quadriceps retards the growth of the medial aspect of the femur, further exacerbating the condition. It is often bilateral in nature and, therefore, can readily be mis--diagnosed or go unnoticed as no gait abnormality or lameness is identified. Traumatic patellar luxation is less common. The most common presentation of a luxating patella is when it dislocates during exercise, causing an irregular gait, often described as skipping. This is noted until the patella spontaneously relocates into the trochlear groove.

A grading system has been developed to measure the severity of patellar luxation, ranging from I to IV. A grade I luxation is an insignificant finding: the patella luxates rarely during normal motion, but can be displaced by digital pressure during a physical examination. A grade IV patellar luxation, however, is one where the patella is permanently displaced and cannot be repositioned, leading to marked deformities of the stifle joint, and an inability to flex or extend the joint. The higher the grade of luxation, the shallower the trochlear groove becomes. The articular surfaces of the patella and trochlea become eroded, leading to an ability to luxate more readily.

The condition inevitably leads over time to the onset of DJD, which may manifest itself in a 'crouching' stance. Prompt identification, assessment, and treatment of the condition are very important to reduce the effects of DJD.

Treatment

In mild cases, physical therapy and massage can create a muscular balance in the pelvic region, especially in the smaller breeds. That can help to stabilize the joint, thereby helping to prevent secondary DJD. Treatment is not quite so straightforward in more severe cases, particularly in larger, heavier dogs. Here, surgery is required to stabilize the joints. Surgical techniques include deepening of the trochlear groove and transposition of the tibial crest, to which the patellar ligament attaches (**193**). The aim of this procedure is to straighten the direction of forces applied between the quadriceps muscle and the patella. Post-surgical rehabilitation by a canine myotherapist is extremely important. Unfortunately, there are cases where the diagnosis has been missed (see Chapter 6).

Cruciate ligament disease

The cruciate ligaments provide stability to the stifle joint, by preventing cranial and caudal movement of the tibia in relation to the femur. As in humans, there are two ligaments within the joint, the cranial and the caudal cruciate ligaments. Cranial cruciate disease is commonly diagnosed within general veterinary practice. The classical history is of a sudden onset of nonweightbearing or toe-touching lame-

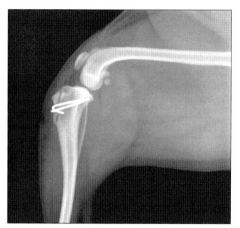

193 Post-surgical radiograph of the stifle of a dog showing K wires used to reattach the tibial crest after its transposition to correct patellar luxation.

ness following exercise; on examination, the limb is seen to be rotated medially. However, as with humans, partial tears, or chronic damage leading to sudden rupture, is also noted, which will not necessarily present with such dramatic and obvious clinical signs. Diseases of the caudal cruciate ligaments are much rarer.

During a physical examination, pain is elicited upon the gentlest palpation of the joint region, and sometimes without flexion and extension. Depending on the duration of clinical signs, a joint swelling (or effusion) can be felt, and compensatory effects, such as contracture of the hamstrings, may be noted (**194**). A technique to evaluate cruciate congruity, known as the drawer test, is undertaken in the conscious animal. This involves manipulating the tibia forwards in relation to the femur, excessive movement being described as 'cranial drawer' (see **176, 177**). However, this is often difficult to assess in the conscious patient, due to the animal's natural reluctance to allow movement of the joint because of the pain caused, not to mention the contracture of the hamstring muscles: the biceps femoris, the semitendinosis, and the semimembranosis. Thus, it is often necessary to undertake examination under sedation or general anaesthesia, at which time confirmatory radiographs are also taken. Classical radiographic changes include joint effusion, compression of the fat pad within the joint, subchondral sclerosis, and osteophyte formation of the trochlear ridge.

Treatment

Surgical treatment is required to stabilize the joint and minimize the development of secondary joint disease. There are many different techniques, from the placement of an extracapsular suture passing from the fabella through a drilled hole in the tibial crest, to a tibial plateau levelling osteotomy (TPLO). The choice depends on the veterinary surgeon's experience and the severity of the disease.

Increasing exercise post-operatively over a period of time, commonly in the region of 6–8 weeks, would be encouraged. Cage rest is rarely required. Post-surgical massage, especially the use of passive movement (see Chapter 6) is required as soon as the surgeon has consented, to manage inappropriate scar tissue and to help gain a good range of movement back to the joint. A return to full function of the limb occurs relatively quickly. Physiotherapy is also usefully employed during the recovery period, to maintain joint flexion and extension, prevent muscle contracture, and speed up the rehabilitation process of muscles that will undoubtedly have become atrophied due to lack of, or abnormal, usage.

Prevention

Possibly, there is a role for myotherapy and massage therapy in preventative care, leading to a more stable and balanced dog with appropriate exercise from puppyhood (see Chapter 3). Continued good exercise management could ensure the stifle is better supported by the gluteal muscles and other deep pelvic supporting muscles (see Chapter 3).

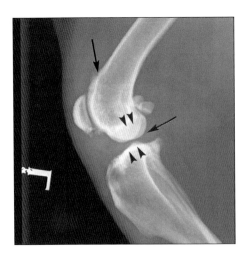

194 Lateral stifle radiograph, showing OA post-cruciate ligament rupture. Note the periosteal new bone in the region of the trochlear ridge (black arrow), effusion or swelling of the joint capsule (arrow), and bone sclerosis (arrowheads).

Disorders of muscles and tendons

Muscular, tendinous, or ligamentous injuries are commonly sustained by animals, but they are often difficult to diagnose unless the traumatic incident has been witnessed by the owner. An experienced practitioner may detect subtle differences in heat which may indicate increased blood supply, possibly indicative of inflammation due to trauma. The fact that muscular injuries are often overlooked is perhaps due to the difficulties that imaging muscular structures presents, and the perceived transient nature of the injury.

Skeletal muscle injury

Injuries to muscle come in two recognized forms, the bruise (contusion) and the strain. The term 'bruise' suggests haemorrhage and muscle fibre disruption as a direct result of trauma, as opposed to a strain, which is defined as stretching or tearing of the groups of fibres, and is perhaps more consistent with abnormal or excessive movement of a muscle beyond its normal range of movement. Muscular injury can cause considerable pain during normal locomotion. Trauma to muscles can result in damage to individual muscle fibres, disruption of the fibril units of muscle, and damage to the vascular supply of the muscle unit, leading to considerable haemorrhage, which further disrupts its continuity. Usually, strains tend to be a little less severe than contusions.

Fortunately, muscle heals readily as it has a very good blood supply. However, this occurs only if the connective tissue surrounding each muscle fibre (the endomysium) remains relatively intact (**195**). If this is not the case, as a result of severe trauma leading to catastrophic haemorrhage, scar or fibrous tissue is laid down, disrupting the normal architecture of the muscle. Scar tissue does not possess the properties of the muscle fibre, i.e. its capability to stretch and contract. Scar tissue, therefore, retards the muscle as a whole, reducing its ability to stretch and contract and, therefore, affecting the motion of the dog.

Muscular injury is invariably caused by trauma, which may or may not be witnessed by the owner. Unlike many orthopaedic diseases, there is no age, breed, or sex predilection.

Treatment

Treatment, if trauma is witnessed, should include the immediate application of a cold compress to the area concerned. The cold compress can take any form, from a specially-designed ice pack to a can of drink! However, the compress, whatever it is, should always be wrapped within a

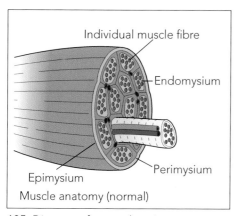

Individual muscle fibre
Endomysium
Perimysium
Epimysium
Muscle anatomy (normal)

195 Diagram of a muscle unit.

towel or similar, to prevent skin trauma as a result of excessive vasoconstriction. For the same reason, a compress should only be applied for short periods of time – not more than 5 minutes – and repeated for as long as the heat persists after the injury (196). If the affected area is superficial, the length of time that the compress is applied should be reduced.

NSAIDs are often administered during the early post-injury period to reduce the inflammation and the pain, although this can often be counterproductive, as the animal automatically feels improvement, moves more readily, and, therefore, does not allow time for healing.

The healing process relies upon the recruitment of mesenchymal cells which migrate to the traumatized area and lay down collagen, forming the initial scar tissue 'scaffold'. This allows future remodelling from one side of the injury to the other. During this time, exercise restriction should be advised, or there may be a replacement of muscle tissue by fibrous tissue, leading to shortening of the muscle and abnormal locomotion. This is an area where physical therapy and massage can help enormously. If trauma is suspected, the dog should be taken as soon as possible to the veterinary surgeon for a diagnosis and quick referral to a therapist. If there is a form of intermittent or difficult to diagnose lameness, the likelihood is there is soft tissue involvement. A good therapist will be able to identify the affected muscle and target the exact area/s requiring treatment. The earlier a therapist can see any dog with muscular trauma, however small, the

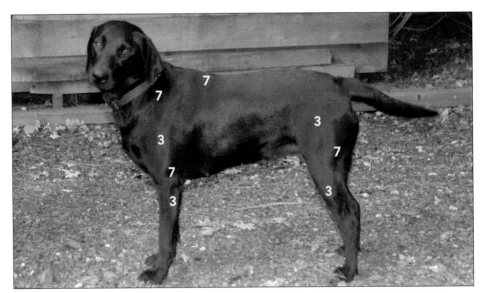

196 Cold compression of muscular trauma. These are the **maximum** times for cold be applied – to be repeated if heat returns. Areas of deep muscle 7 minutes, areas of superficial bone 3 minutes; do not exceed these times.

better and quicker the recovery will be, and fewer secondary compensatory issues will have time to develop. Correct massage techniques will enable scar tissue to be broken down and fibre alignment re-established, maintaining a balanced muscular system (see Chapter 6).

Tendon rupture

It is not uncommon for penetrating injuries to the superficial structures of the limbs, poorly protected by muscle units to result in partial or complete rupture of a tendon. Chronic, extreme overextension of a tendon may produce a similar outcome. Diagnosis is relatively straight-forward: the lacerated tendon ends can often be observed through the skin wound, or the diagnosis can be made following debridement under anaesthesia.

Treatment

Treatment is invariably surgical, with appositional and deep supporting sutures both being used to facilitate healing (**197**). The healing process is similar to that of muscle, but slower, as the blood supply is poorer. It is very important to coapt the limb after surgery for up to 3 weeks, by which time considerable atrophy of the associated muscle groups will have occurred. Carefully managed physical therapy and massage can help to assist the primary and secondary, compensatory muscular conditions.

Neoplasia

Neoplasia, the formation of 'new and abnormal growth, specifically in which cell multiplication is uncontrolled and progressive', is a well-recognized cause of lameness in the dog. Neoplasia can technically stem from any cell of the body, including the bones, joints, and any of their constituent parts.

The most commonly diagnosed bone tumour is osteosarcoma, which accounts for 90% of long bone tumours in large and giant breed dogs. Osteosarcoma is an aggressive neoplasm, invariably meta-

stasizing in the early stages of the disease process. The most common sites for this particular neoplasm are the metaphyseal regions of the long bones, at the proximal

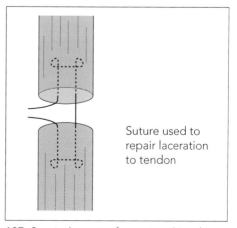

Suture used to repair laceration to tendon

197 Surgical repair of a ruptured **tendon**.

humerus, distal radius, distal femur and proximal tibia (**198**), away from the elbow and at the knee. It is postulated that wear and tear, excessive load, and genetics may play a part in the disease.

Osteosarcoma is locally invasive, causing an intense periosteal reaction in conjunction with lysis or erosion of the cortex. This renders the bone weak, and prone to pathological fracture. The condition is known to be extremely painful and, due to its rapid progression and metastasis, the prognosis is grave. Diagnosis is tentatively made by palpation and radiographs (**199**, **200**); the disease differs from severe OA as it does not cross from one bone to another. It is imperative that a physiotherapy practitioner be aware that, should a prominent bony swelling be palpated, at any of the aforementioned predilection sites, immediate consultation with a veterinary surgeon is required.

Treatment
Treatment is usually palliative; amputation, limb sparing, bisphosphonate medication, and chemotherapy are often instigated in an attempt to prolong life. To assist any secondary muscular problems, carefully managed physiotherapy and massage can help enormously.

Spinal disease
Several disease processes of the spine arise in dogs. Pathologies of note include discospondylitis (infection of the intervertebral disc and the adjacent vertebrae), intervertebral disc disease (displacement of the intervertebral disc, leading to spinal cord trauma of varying severity), chronic disc degeneration (**201**), spondylosis deformans (see later), and neoplasia. It should be emphasized that if a dog is being treated by a physical therapist and spinal disease is suspected, physiotherapeutic treatment should be halted and veterinary advice sought immediately. Such cases should only be treated under strict veterinary supervision.

Treatment
The treatment of choice in many circumstances involving vertebral trauma, intervertebral disc disease, and spinal cord trauma will involve surgery and a prolonged post-operative recovery period. It is, therefore, highly likely that a physiotherapy practitioner would be involved in a post-surgical rehabilitation programme of some kind during their professional career. Certain situations exist, however, where surgery may be deemed inappropriate, due to the age of the patient, or the

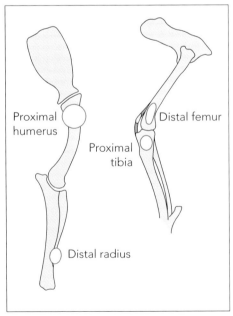

Proximal humerus

Distal femur

Proximal tibia

Distal radius

198 Predilection sites for osteosarcoma.

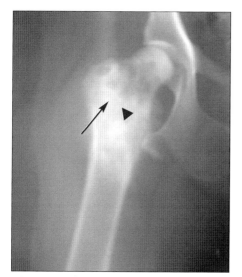

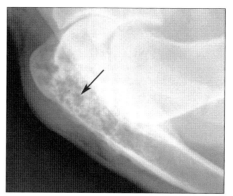

200 Lateral radiograph of the elbow showing osteosarcoma of the proximal ulna. Note the areas of bone lysis and destruction of the cortex (arrow).

199 Ventrodorsal radiograph of the hip of a dog showing osteosarcoma of the proximal femur. Note the periosteal new bone (arrow) and bone lysis within the cortex of the femur (arrow head).

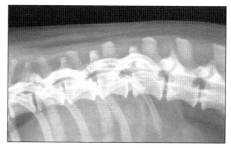

201 Radiograph showing calcification of the intervertebral disc.

owner's financial constraints, e.g. in cases of chronic disc degeneration or disc disease (types 1 and 2). The physiotherapy practitioner may, in such circumstances, be asked to provide crucial conservative treatment to maintain the quality of life of the affected animal by ensuring a reasonable level of movement, and preserving mobility for as long as possible. Treatment should be specifically designed for the region of the spine affected (cervical, thoracic, lumbar).

Spondylosis deformans

Spondylosis is defined as the formation of bony 'spurs' on the vertebrae, often leading to fusion of an intervertebral joint, resulting in ankylosis (**202, 203**). It is often seen as an incidental finding when thoracic or abdominal radiography is undertaken. It is a chronic condition of older animals and is typified by osteogenesis and osteophyte formation at the dorsal margins of the vertebrae. Spondylosis is usually of no clinical importance, although, in some circumstances, pain (thought to be similar to that of arthritis) is noted. Clinical signs including difficulty to rise, reluctance to climb or jump, and exercise intolerance.

Treatment

There is no specific treatment, but physiotherapy and massage may help in clinically affected cases. However, the effects of massage therapy are dependent on the position and the extent of the spondylytic lesion. This can be a frustrating condition for the physiotherapist to treat, as the response can vary from excellent to exceedingly disappointing. However, like all lameness issues, therapists most certainly have a role in assisting the secondary muscular conditions.

Degenerative myelopathy

Degenerative myelopathy, otherwise known as chronic degenerative radiculomyelopathy (CDRM) is a degenerative disorder of the white matter of the spinal cord, involving the demyelination (stripping of the myelin sheath) of nerve fibres, designed to accelerate nerve impulses. The cause of CDRM remains unclear; however, theories include an immune-mediated cause, breeding, or nutritional deficiencies. The initial clinical signs include a seemingly innocuous weakness of the pelvic limbs, progressing to the classical sign of scuffed shortened nails and knuckling of the pelvic limbs as proprioceptive deficits progress (see **42**). Often an increased muscular tone, particularly in the quadriceps group, is evident, and reflexes are generally exaggerated, suggesting a lack of nerve impulse inhibition. This narrows the region of suspicion to the upper motor neuron system, and particularly spinal cord segments T3–L3. Diagnostic imaging is largely unremarkable; therefore, diagnosis relies on the clinical signs and the exclusion of other diseases, such as spinal trauma and intervertebral disc disease.

Treatment

Treatment regimes used to date have proved ineffective. Steroids or immune-modulating drugs aimed at nullifying any immune-mediated condition have proved ineffectual. Other treatments concentrate on the nutritional aetiology of the disease. Neither appears to halt the progression of the condition. Nevertheless, myotherapy and massage can assist enormously with the compensatory muscular results of this extremely distressing condition; this is especially relevant in the lumbar region and the shoulders. Because this condition leads to large pelvic limb proprioceptive deficits, the shoulder muscles become hypertonic and engorged from pulling the dog forwards; by easing the shoulders, this can be diminished, and mobility assisted. The lumbar region is under huge stress to remain stable; therefore, easing pain in the area can also help mobility, and, more importantly, quality of life.

Peripheral neurological disease

Neurological deficits causing lameness in the dog are usually due to spinal cord disease; these have already been discussed. However, lameness may also be due to peripheral nerve disease, which can be caused by trauma, neoplasia, or degeneration. The effects vary according to the severity of the damage and the point of injury or disease. As before, there is no specific treatment, but symptomatic physiotherapy and massage can be very helpful.

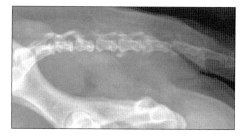

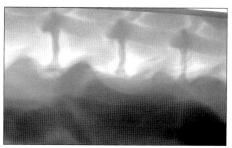

202, 203 Lateral radiograph of the lumbar spine showing a spondylytic lesion in the coccygeal (**202**) and lumbar (**203**) vertebrae.

Glossary of Terms

Miscellaneous definitions

Canine exercise Physiology (Galen Natural Progression): a method of assessment and maximizing movement through natural exercises.

Golgi tendon organ: specialized organ within the tendon that reports on the tension or force being exerted through the muscle to the tendon.

Myotherapy: a specialized therapy that accurately assesses and treats muscle pain and enhances muscle function.

Neuromuscular junction (NMJ): the junction of a motor neuron axon terminal with the motor end plate on a muscle; it is where movement is initiated.

Organelle: a specialized subunit within a cell with a specific role, such as mitochondria, which generate most of the cell's supply of adenosine triphosphate (ATP), which is a source of energy. They are found in many cell types, but are most numerous within muscle cells.

Proprioception: the sense that indicates where the various parts of the body are located in relation to each other.

Reciprocal inhibition: the mechanism whereby the antagonist (muscle) relaxes while the agonist (muscle) contracts, and vice versa.

Prefixes

A, a – without, lack of, e.g. ataxia
Ab – away, e.g. abduction
Ad – towards, e.g. adduction
Ana – apart, e.g. anatomy (taking apart)
Ante – before, in front of, forward, e.g. anteflex (bend forward)
Anti – against, opposing, e.g. antibrachii
Auto – self, e.g. autoimmune, automatic
Bi – two
Circum – around
Dia – between, through, apart, across, e.g. diameter, diaphragm
Dis – apart from, free from, e.g. dissect

Ecto – outer
Exo – exterior, e.g. exoskeleton
End/endo/ent/ento – within, inner, e.g. endoscope
Extra/extro – outside, e.g. extracurricular, extrinsic
Hyper – extra, e.g. hypertrophy, hyperglycaemic
Hypo – below, deficient, e.g. hypodermic (beneath the skin)
Infra – behind, below, e.g. infraspinatus
Inter – between, e.g. intercostals
Intra – within, e.g. intravenous
Intro – into, within, e.g. introversion, introduction
Meso – middle, e.g. mesoderm (middle cell layer)
Meta – change, e.g. metamorphosis
Multi – many
Neo – new
Para – beside, beyond, after
Peri – around, e.g. periosteum
Poly – many
Post – after
Pre/pro – before
Re – again, backwards, e.g. retract
Retro – behind
Semi – half
Sub – below
Supra/super – above, e.g. supraspinatus
Sym/syn – together, with, e.g. symbiotic, synapse
Trans – across, through
Ultra – beyond, excess

Suffixes

-oma – tumour, e.g. carcinoma (malignant tumour)
-ac,-al, -ic, -oux, -tic -ous – pertaining to, relating to, e.g. thoracic, tarsal
-algia, -dynia – pain, e.g. neuralgia
-ectomy,– removal, e.g. appendectomy
-aemia – blood, e.g. leukaemia, anaemia
-ent, -er, -ist, -or – person or agent, e.g. anatomist
-esis, -ia, -iasis, -ism, -ity, -osis, -sis, -tion, -y – state or condition, e.g. lordosis

-form – resembling, shaped like, e.g. fusiform

-itis – inflammation, e.g. arthritis, neuritis, dermatitis

-logy – study of

-penia/paenia – deficiency, lack of

-stomy – surgical opening e.g. colostomy

Skeletal terminology

Crest – a ridge of bone, e.g. the occipital crest

Condyle – a rounded projection of bone at a joint, e.g. the femoral condyles

Epicondyle – a separate prominence close to the condyle

Foramen – a natural opening in a bone, through which nerves, blood vessels, and so on pass, e.g. the obturator foramen of the pelvis

Fossa – a hollow or depression, e.g. the olecranon fossa of the elbow

Head – a rounded articular surface, e.g. the head of the femur

Tuberocity – a protuberance of a bone, e.g. the tibial tuberocity

Trochanter – a large rough process of the femur

Trochlea – a depression in the bone where major tendons lie, e.g. the trochlear groove of the knee joint

Tubercle – a rounded process where a muscle inserts, e.g. the greater tubercle of the femur

Muscle names

Externus – outer

Gracilis – slender

Latissimus – wide

Longissimus – long

Quadratus – square

Rectus – straight

Rhomboideus – kite, diamond-shaped

Scalenus – unequal, irregular triangle

Serratus – saw-tooth

Teres – round or cylindrical

Transversus – across

Vastus – great

Derivation of muscle names

Action, e.g. extensor carpi radialis, adductor

Direction of fibres, e.g. orbicular or obliques

Location, e.g. external obliques

Number of sections or heads, e.g. triceps

Origin, insertion, e.g. sternomandibulus

Shape, e.g. rhomboideus

Movement definitions

Abduct – move away from the midline of the body

Adduct – move towards the midline of the body

Circumduct – move circularly or conically e.g. a function of the coxofemoral (hip) joint

Depress – draw downwards

Elevate – draw upwards

Extend – increasing the inner angle of the joint, arch the back dorsally (Hyperextension is when a joint extends beyond 180°.)

Flex – decrease the inner angle of the joint, arch the back upwards

Laterally flex – bend sideways, e.g. turning head and neck

Laterally rotate – rotate outwards

Medially rotate – rotate inwards

Pronate – rotate the lateral aspect of the paw medially

Protract – draw forward

Retract – draw backwards

Supinate – rotate the lateral aspect of the paw laterally (the normal position of the paw is supine)

Anatomical positioning of muscles

Extrinsic muscles are those that attach the appendicular skeleton (limbs) to the axial skeleton (torso).

Intrinsic muscles are those that attach to the appendicular skeleton but not to the axial, or those that attach to the axial skeleton and not to the appendicular skeleton.

Axial muscles are divided into two groups:

Epaxial – muscles that lie dorsal to the transverse processes and are involved with extension of the vertebral column.

Hypaxial – all muscles that lie ventral to the transverse processes of the vertebrae, including the abdominal and thoracic walls.

Muscle roles

Agonist or prime mover – muscle whose contraction causes a specific movement.

Antagonist – muscle which contracts in opposition to the agonist.

Fixator – muscles which stabilize an area for the action of the agonist, e.g. the fixator muscles of the scapula (e.g. m. supraspinatus) and form a firm foundation for movement within the distal thoracic limb.

Reciprocal inhibition – neural inhibition response causing relaxation of the antagonist when the agonist contracts, thus allowing easy movement without any opposing tension.

Synergist – these tend to be the smaller, deeper muscles that work with the agonist to provide isolation and stability to a joint.

Types of muscle movements

Concentric contraction – contraction of muscle fibres in which they are shortened; this is used in protraction, retraction, adduction, and abduction.

Eccentric contraction – lengthening of the muscle fibres under tension, when forces cause the muscle to extend even though the muscle fibres themselves are shortening. Therefore, the muscle develops tension while lengthening, e.g. when landing after a jump, the antagonist contracts, thereby stabilizing the movement.

Isometric contraction – muscle fibres contracting against a fixed resistance in order to provide stability, e.g. when the dog is standing still on a moving platform.

Planes of motion

A plane, here, is an imaginary flat area bisecting the dog's body (**56**):

- Frontal plane – divides the body horizontally into upper and lower halves.
- Sagittal plane – divides the body vertically into left and right halves.
- Transverse plane – divides the body vertically into cranial and caudal halves.

Regions of the body

Caudal – part that is nearest to the tail.

Cranial – part that is nearest to the head.

Distal – part that is furthest away from the body or organ.

Dorsal – the upper surface of the body or the front surface of the carpus and tarsus.

Palmar – bottom surface of the thoracic limb paw.

Plantar – bottom surface of the pelvic limb paw.

Proximal – part that is nearest to the body or organ.

Rostral – in the head, the part that is closest to the nose.

Ventral – lower surface of the body. This is not used in the limbs, where the terms palmar (front legs) or plantar (back legs) are used.

Regions of the limbs

Antebrachium – part of the thoracic limb between the elbow and the carpus.

Brachium – part of the thoracic limb between the shoulder and the elbow.

Crus – part of the pelvic limb between the stifle and the tarsus.

Manus – distal part of the thoracic limb (includes the carpus, the metacarpus, and the digits).

Pes – distal part of the pelvic limb (includes the tarsus, the metatarsus, and digits).

Further Reading

Coughlan AR, Miller A (eds) (1998). *BSAVA Manual of Small Animal Fracture Repair and Management*. British Small Animal Veterinary Association. ISBN 978-0905214375.

De Domenico G (2007). *Beard's Massage – Principles and Practice of Soft Tissue Manipulation*. WB Saunders/Elsevier, 5th edn. ISBN 978-0721603506.

Fischer MS, Lilje KE (2011). *Dogs in Motion*. VDH Service GmbH und Franckh-Kosmos Verlags-GmbH & Co. ISBN 978-3981433906.

Hodges PW, Richardson CA (1996). Inefficient muscular stabilization of the lumbar spine associated with low back pain. *Spine* **21**: 2640–50.

Myers TW (2008). *Anatomy Trains. Myofascial Meridians for Manual and Movement Therapists*, 2nd edn. Churchill Livingstone. ISBN 978-0443102837.

Robertson J (2010). *The Complete Dog Massage Manual*. Veloce Publishing Ltd. ISBN 978-1845843229.

Robertson J, Pope E (2011). *Exercising Your Puppy: a Natural and Gentle Approach*. Veloce Publishing Ltd. ISBN 978-1845843229.

Robertson J, Pope E (2012). From Tongue to Tail: the Integrated Movement of the Dog (DVD). Parkes Publication.

Whalen-Shaw PW (2000). *Canine Massage – The Workbook*. Bookmasters Inc. ISBN 978-1930511026.

Wyche S (2002). *The Horse's Muscles in Motion*. Crowood Press. ISBN 978-1861264565.

Appendix

The muscles of the dog – their placement and actions

Extrinsic muscles of the thoracic limb				
Muscle	**Origin**	**Insertion**	**Innervation**	**Action**
Trapezius (Protractor and retractor of scapula) (204, 210)	Dorsal median raphe (seam) of the neck and the supraspinous ligament from the level of the 3rd cervical vertebrae to the level of the spinous processes of the 9th/10th vertebrae	Cervical part – dorsal two-thirds of the scapula spine Thoracic part – dorsal third of the scapula spine	Dorsal branch of accessory nerve (XI)	Cervical part – draws scapula craniodorsally Thoracic part – draws scapula caudodorsally Cervical & thoracic parts acting together – draw scapula dorsally
Omo-transversarius (Lateral flexor of neck, aids protraction of thoracic limb) (204, 207)	Acromion of scapula (caudally)	Wing of atlas (cranially)	Ventral branch of 4th cervical nerve	Draws scapula and thoracic limb forwards Flexes neck laterally
Rhomboideus (Thoracic limb stabilizer and elevator of scapula) (205, 208, 219)	Rhomboideus capitis – nuchal crest of the occipital bone Rhomboideus cervicis – dorsal median raphe of the neck from the 2nd cervical to 1st thoracic vertebra Rhomboideus thoracis – spinous processes of the first seven thoracic vertebrae	Capitis – cranial dorsal border of scapula Cervicis – caudal (base) of scapula, medially and laterally Thoracis – caudal (base) of scapula, medially and laterally	Ventral branches of cervical and thoracic spinal nn.	Elevates and retracts thoracic limb Draws scapula against trunk When neck is lowered, elevates neck

(continues)

Extrinsic muscles of the thoracic limb (continued)

Muscle	Origin	Insertion	Innervation	Action
Serratus Ventralis (Supports trunk and thoracic limb) (209, 219)	Serratus cervicis – transverse processes of the last five cervical vertebrae Serratus thoracis – first seven or eight ribs ventral to their midline	Dorsomedial third of the serrated surface of scapula	Ventral rami of cervical spinal nn. and long thoracic nerve	Most important muscle supporting the trunk Carries trunk and shoulder forward and back Depresses scapula
Sternohyoideus	Manubrium of sternum	Basihyoideum	Ventral branch of first cervical nerve	Draws the tongue caudally (when hypertonic could have negative influence on balance)
Brachiocephalicus (Prime shoulder extensor) (204, 206)	Cleidobrachialis – ventral aspect of clavicular intersection Cleidocephalicus – dorsal aspect of clavicular intersection	Cleidobrachialis – distal third, cranial surface of humerus Cleidocephalicus cervical part – cranial half, mid dorsal fibrous raphe and occasionally to nuchal crest of occipital bone Cleidomastoideus – mastoid part of temporal bone	Accessory nerve and ventral branches of cervical spinal nn.	Cleidobrachialis – extends shoulder joint and advances thoracic limb Cleidocephalicus – draws head to the side and extends neck
Latissimus dorsi (Prime shoulder flexor) (204, 215, 219)	Thoracolumbar fascia from spinous processes of most caudal seven or eight thoracic vertebrae and lumbar vertebrae; most caudal to or four ribs	Teres major tuberosity of humerus and teres major tendon	Thoracodorsal nerve	Prime flexor of shoulder joint When limb is fixed – draws the trunk cranially When limb is free – draws the limb caudally

(continues)

Extrinsic muscles of the thoracic limb (continued)

Muscle	Origin	Insertion	Innervation	Action
Superficial pectoral (Thoracic limb adductor) (218)	Transverse portion – the first two or three sternabrae Descending portion - manubrium	All but the most distal part of the crest of the greater tubercle of the humerus	Cranial pectoral nerve	Adducts limb when non weightbearing Prevents limb from abducting when weightbearing
Deep pectoral (Thoracic limb adductor and retractor) (218)	Manubrium of sternum and the fibrous raphe between fellow muscles The deep abdominal fascia in the region of the xiphoid cartilage (the caudal end of the sternum)	Major portion – partly muscular, partly tendinous on the lesser tubercle of the humerus Also via an aponeurosis to the greater tubercle and its crest Lesser portion – medial brachial fascia	Caudal pectoral nerve	Adducts the limb when limb advanced and fixed – pulls trunk cranially and to extend the shoulder joint When limb non weight bearing – draws limb caudally and flexes shoulder joint

Intrinsic muscles of thoracic limb

Muscle	Origin	Insertion	Innervation	Action
Deltoideus (Shoulder abduction Aids thoracic limb flexion) (204, 217)	Spinous head – scapular spine, blending with the infraspinatus	Deltoid tuberosity of the humerus	Axillary nerve	Spinous head – flexes shoulder Acromial head – abducts shoulder
Supraspinatus (Shoulder extensor and stabilizer) (216, 219, 221)	Acromial head – acromion Supraspinous fossa of scapula	Cranially on the greater tubercle of the humerus by means of a thick tendon	Suprascapular nerve	Extends shoulder Stabilizes and prevents dislocation of shoulder
Infraspinatus (Shoulder flexor) (216, 219, 221)	Infraspinous fossa and spine of scapula	Lateral side of greater tubercle of humerus	Suprascapular nerve	Flexes shoulder Abducts shoulder Stabilizes shoulder
Coracobrachialis (Shoulder extensor and adductor) (216, 219)	Coracoid process of scapula	Caudomedial area of proximal humerus	Musculo-cutaneous nerve	Extends shoulder Adducts shoulder Stabilizes shoulder joint
Triceps brachii (Shoulder flexor and elbow extensor) (204, 214, 219)	Long head – caudal border of scapula Lateral head – tricipital line of humerus Accessory head – caudal neck of humerus Medial head – crest of lesser tubercle near the teres major tuberosity of humerus	Olecranon process	Radial nerve	Extends elbow joint Helps tense antebrachial fascia Long head – flexes shoulder joint
Biceps brachii (Shoulder extensor and elbow flexor) (212, 219)	Supraglenoid tubercle of scapula	Radial tuberosity, proximomedial ulna	Musculo-cutaneous nerve	Flexes elbow Extends shoulder Some passive stability when weightbearing, preventing shoulder flexion
Brachialis (Elbow flexor) (211, 212)	Proximal third, lateral surface of humerus	Ulnar and radial tuberosities	Musculo-cutaneous nerve	Flexes elbow

(continues)

Intrinsic muscles of thoracic limb (continued)

EPAXIAL MUSCLES (220, 221)
This group of dorsal vertebral and costal muscles are divided into three individual muscle groups lying in parallel, each overlapping. It is almost impossible to give exact insertions and origins, due to the many overlapping fascicles
Extensors of the vertebral column dorsally, and, when unilaterally contracted, laterally
Deep and medial:
Transversospinalis system: spinalis, semispinalis, multifidus, rotators, interspinalis, and interansversarius (complex that joins vertebrae – both those adjacent and slightly distal)
Intermediate portion:
Longissimus capitis – origin T1–3; insertion: mastoid part of temporal bone (passing over atlas)
Longissimus cervicis – lying in an overlapping style in the angle of the cervical and thoracic vertebrae and inserting on the transverse processes of C4–7
Longissimus thoracis and longissimus lumborum – originate from crest of ilium via aponeurosis to spinous processes of lumbar and thoracic vertebrae
The most ventrally situated of the group:
Iliocostalis thoracis – origin transverse process of C7–C12
Iliocostalis lumborum – origin wing of ilium and then on the transverse processes of lumbar vertebrae and the last four to five costals

---

Muscles of the head and neck

Muscle	Origin	Insertion	Innervation	Action
Masseter (204)	Zygomatic arch	Masseteric fossa of mandible	Mandibular nerve (branch of the trigeminal nerve)	Raises the mandible (closes the jaw)
Sternocephalicus (204)	Manubrium	Mastoid part of temporal bone and nuchal crest of occipital bone	Accessory nerve and ventral branches of cervical spinal nerve	Draws head and neck to the side
Splenius (206, 220, 221)	Cranial border of thoracolumbar fascia Spines of first three thoracic vertebrae Entire median raphe of neck	Nuchal crest and mastoid part of temporal bone	Dorsal branch of cervical and thoracic nerve.	Extension and lateral flexion of head and neck

Muscles of the pelvic limb: caudal thigh muscles (hamstrings)

Muscle	Origin	Insertion	Innervation	Action
Biceps femoris (Hip, stifle and tarsus extensor Stifle flexor Pelvic limb retractor) **(222)**	Sacrotuberous ligament and ischiatic tuberosity	Patellar ligament and cranial border of tibia via fascia lata and crural fascia Tibial body via crural fascia Calcaneal tuberosity	Sciatic nerve Cranial part receives additional stimulation from the caudal gluteal nerve	Extends hip, stifle, and tarsus Caudal part of muscle flexes the stifle Retracts pelvic limb
Semi-membranosus (Hip extensor and stifle flexor) **(222, 227, 228)**	Ischiatic tuberosity	Distal medial lip of caudal rough surface of femur Proximal medial surface of tibia (medial tibial condyle)	Sciatic nerve	Extends hip Femoral attachment extends stifle Tibial attachment flexes or extends stifle depending on position of limb
Semi-tendinosus (Hip and hock extensor Stifle flexor) **(222, 227–229)**	Ischiatic tuberosity	Distocranial border of tibia Medial surface, body of tibia The tuber calcanei by means of the crural fascia	Sciatic nerve	Extends hip Flexes stifle Extends hock

Medial thigh muscles

Muscle	Origin	Insertion	Innervation	Action
Sartorius (Hip flexor) (226, 227, 229)	Cranial part – iliac crest and thoracolumbar fascia Caudal part – cranioventral iliac spine and adjacent ventral border of ilium	Cranial part – patella Caudal part – cranial border of tibia	Femoral nerve	Flexes the hip Cranial part – extends stifle Caudal part – flexes stifle
Gracilis (Limb adductor) (226, 229)	Pelvic symphysis by means of symphysial tendon	Cranial border of tibia (and with the semitendinosis), the tuber calcanei	Obturator nerve	Adducts pelvic limb Flexes stifle Extends hip and hock
Pectineus (Limb adductor and hip flexor) (226, 228, 229)	Iliopubic eminence	Medial lip, caudal rough surface (facies aspera) of femur	Obturator nerve	Adducts pelvic limb Flexes hip
Adductor (Limb adductor and hip extensor) (228, 229)	Entire pelvic symphysis by means of the symphysial tendon, the adjacent part of the ischiatic arch, and ventral surface of the pubis and ischium	Entire lateral lip of caudal facies aspera (rough face of femur)	Obturator nerve	Adducts pelvic limb Extends hip

Lateral thigh muscles

Muscle	Origin	Insertion	Innervation	Action
Tensor fascia latae (Hip flexor and stifle extensor) (222)	Tuber coxae and adjacent part of ilium Aponeurosis of middle gluteal muscle	Cranial superficial part – patella and tibial tuberosity by means of the fascia lata and patella ligament Caudal deeper part – lateral lip of facies aspera of the femur	Cranial gluteal nerve	Flexes hip Extends stifle Tensor of the fascia lata Draws limb forward in cranial movement of the stride
Superficial gluteal (Hip extensor and limb abductor) (222, 224)	Lateral border of sacrum and first caudal vertebra, partly by means of the sacrotuberous ligament Cranial dorsal iliac spine by way of gluteal fascia	Third trochanter of femur	Caudal gluteal nerve	Extends hip Abducts pelvic limb
Middle gluteal (Hip extensor and abductor) (222, 224)	Crest and gluteal surface of ilium	Greater trochanter of femur	Cranial gluteal nerve	Extends and abduct hip Rotates pelvic limb medially Aids stabilization within coxofemoral joint
Deep gluteal (Hind limb extensor and abductor) (224)	Body of ilium and sciatic spine	Cranial aspect of greater trochanter	Cranial gluteal nerve	Extends and abducts pelvic limb Rotates pelvic limb medially

Sublumbar muscles

Muscle	Origin	Insertion	Innervation	Action
Iliopsoas (Hip flexor) (223, 225)	Psoas major – transverse processes of lumbar vertebrae Iliacus – ventral surface of ilium	Psoas major – lesser trochanter, with iliacus Iliacus – lesser trochanter with iliacus	Ventral branches of lumbar spinal nn.	Flexes hip Flexes vertebral column Extends lumbar spine When pelvic limb is extended, draws limb forward Supinates hip When limb fixed, stabilizes vertebral column Flexes hip
Quadratus lumborum (Lateral flexor of the vertebrae)	Last three thoracic and lumbar transverse processes	Transverse processes of the cranial lumbar vertebrae and auricular surface of the pelvis	Ventral branches of the lumbar spinal nn.	Lateral flexion and fixation of the lumbar vertebral column

Femoral muscles

Muscle	Origin	Insertion	Innervation	Action
Quadriceps femoris (Major stifle extensor) (227, 228, 229)	Rectus femoris – ilium Vasti muscles: Vastus lateralis – lateral side and proximal end of femur Vastus intermedius – lateral side and proximal end of femur Vastus medialis – medial side, proximal end, and cranial surface of femur	All four bellies of the quadriceps femoris form one common tendon of insertion which extends distally to invest the patella and insert on the tibial tuberosity	Femoral nerve	Extends stifle Flexes hip (rectus femoris only)

Deep muscles of the coxofemoral joint

Muscle	Origin	Insertion	Innervation	Action
Internal obturator	Symphysis of the pelvis and dorsal surface of the ischium and pubis	Trochanteric fossa of the femur	Sciatic nerve	Rotates the pelvic limb laterally at coxofemoral joint
Gemelli	Lateral surface of the ischium caudal to the acetabulum	Trochanteric fossa	Sciatic nerve	Rotates the pelvic limb laterally at coxofemoral joint
Quadratus femoris	Ventral surface of the caudal part of the ischium	Trochanteric fossa	Sciatic nerve	Rotates the pelvic limb and extends the hip
External obturator	Ventral surface of the pubis and ischium	Trochanteric fossa	Obturator nerve	Rotates hip laterally
Articularis coxae	Lunate surface of acetabulum	Proximal and medial to the line of vastus lateralis		Flexes the hip

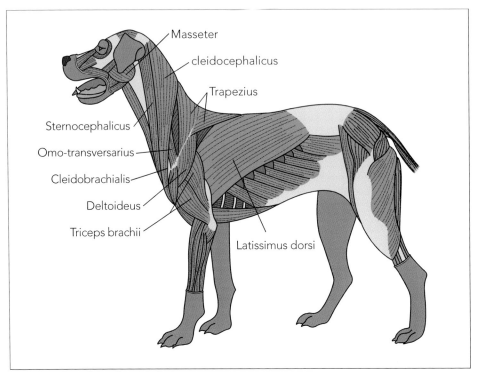

204 Muscles of the thoracic limb.

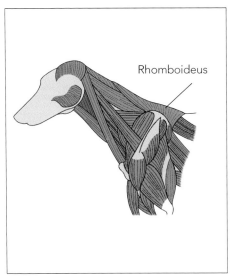

205 Rhomboideus.

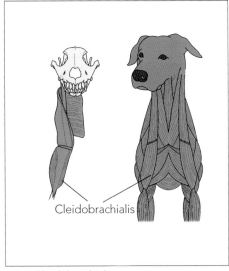

206 Cleidobrachialis.

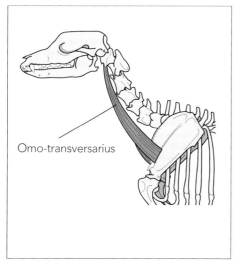

207 Omo-transversarius.

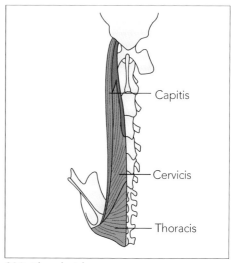

208 Rhomboideus.

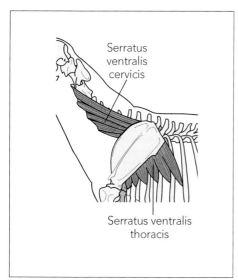

209 Serratus ventralis.

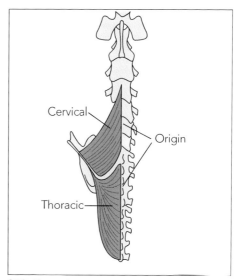

210 Trapezius.

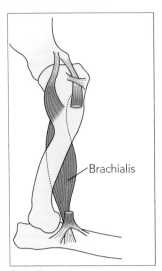

211 Trapezius

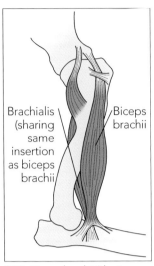

212 Biceps brachii (sharing same insertion as biceps brachii

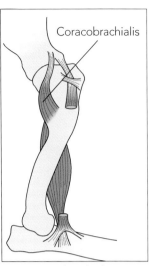

213 Coracobrachialis

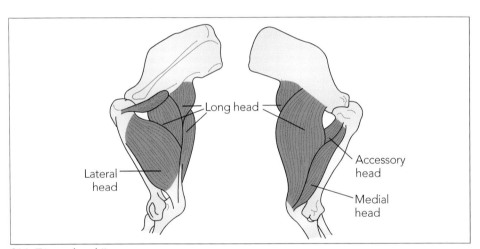

214 Triceps brachii

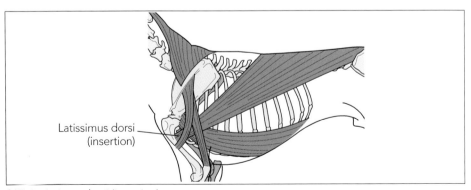

215 Latissimus dorsi (insertion).

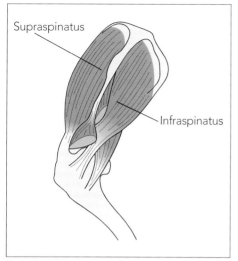

216 Supraspinatus, Infraspinatus.

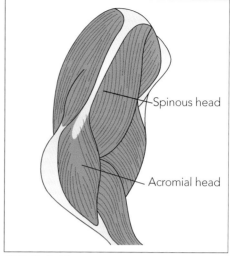

217 Deltoideus.

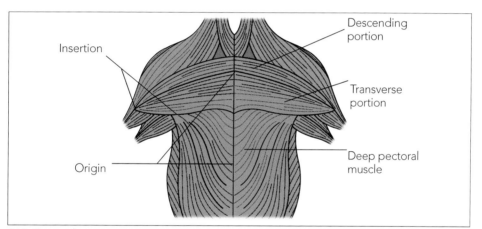

218 Pectoral group.

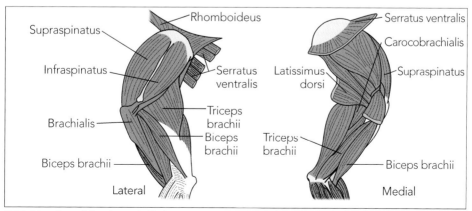

219 Muscles of the thoracic limb.

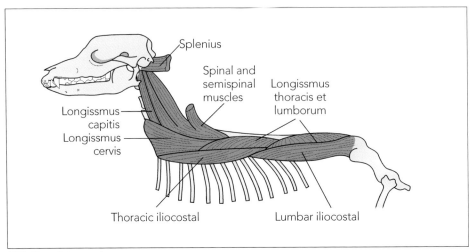

220 Epaxial muscles.

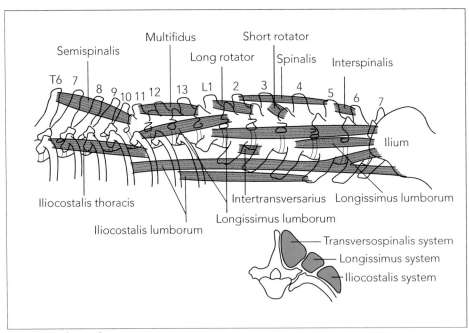

221 Epaxial muscles.

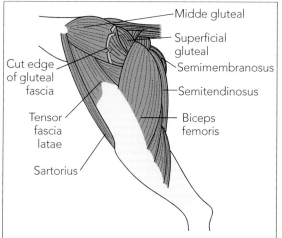

222 Muscles of the pelvic limb.

223 Sublumber muscles.

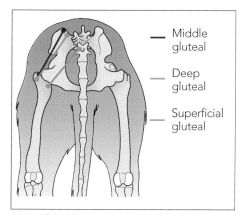

224 Gluteal muscles.

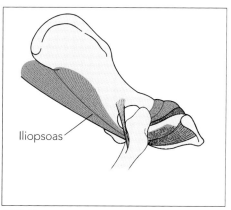

225 Iliopsoas.

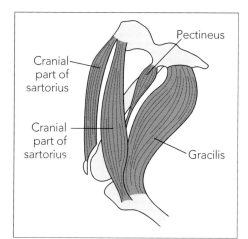

226 Medial thigh muscles.

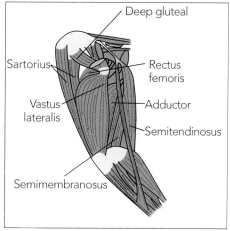

227 Femoral muscles.

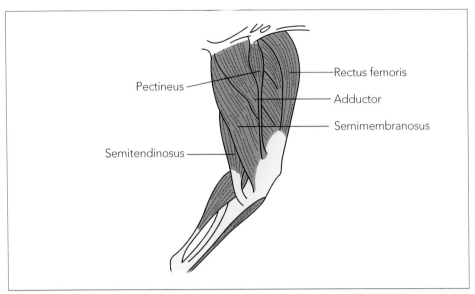

228 Muscles of the pelvic limb.

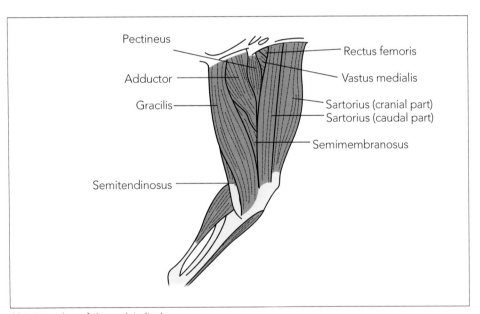

229 Muscles of the pelvic limb.

Index